Infection Control Compliance Guide: Understanding the JCAHO's Standards

Gail Bennett, RN, MSN, CIC

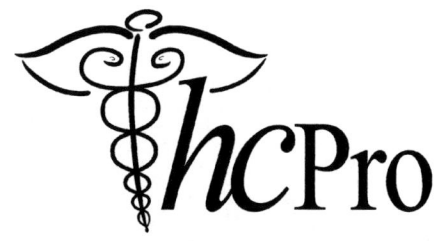

Infection Control Compliance Guide: Understanding the JCAHO's Standards is published by HCPro, Inc.

Copyright 2004 by HCPro, Inc.

All rights reserved. Printed in the United States of America.   5   4   3   2   1

ISBN 1-57839-466-X

No part of this publication may be reproduced, in any form or by any means, without prior written consent of HCPro, Inc., or the Copyright Clearance Center (978/750-8400). Please notify us immediately if you have received an unauthorized copy.

HCPro, Inc., provides information resources for the healthcare industry.

HCPro, Inc., is not affiliated in any way with the Joint Commission on Accreditation of Healthcare Organizations, which owns the JCAHO trademark.

Gail Bennett, RN, MSN, CIC, Author
Judith Kelliher, Senior Managing Editor
Lauren Rubenzahl, Copy Editor
Susan Darbyshire, Layout Artist
Jackie Diehl Singer, Graphic Artist
Shane Katz, Cover Designer
Jean St. Pierre, Creative Director
Bob Croce, Group Publisher
Suzanne Perney, Publisher

Advice given is general. Readers should consult professional counsel for specific legal, ethical, or clinical questions. Arrangements can be made for quantity discounts.

For more information, contact:

HCPro, Inc.
P.O. Box 1168
Marblehead, MA 01945
Telephone: 800/650-6787 or 781/639-1872
Fax: 800/639-8511 or 781/639-2982
E-mail: *customerservice@hcpro.com*

Visit HCPro, Inc., at its World Wide Web site:
www.hcpro.com

Contents

About the author vii

How to use this book viii
    Chapter summaries viii

Introduction x
    Overview of 2005 standards x
    Compliance and beyond xi
    References xiii

Chapter One: Organization-wide IC program 1
    An organization-wide IC program is implemented 2
    Individuals and/or positions with the authority to take steps to prevent or control the acquisition
        and transmission of infectious agents are identified 2
    All applicable organization components and functions are integrated into the IC program 5
    Systems are in place to communicate with licensed independent practitioners (LIP),
        staff, students/trainees, volunteers, and, as appropriate, visitors and patients about infection
        prevention and control issues, including their responsibilities in preventing
        the spread of infection within the hospital 5
    The hospital has systems for reporting identified infections 5
    Systems for investigating outbreaks of infectious diseases are in place 7
    Applicable policies and procedures are in place throughout the hospital 13
    The hospital has a written IC plan 13

Introduction to chapters two, three, four, and five 23

Chapter Two: Risks for acquisition and transmission of infectious agents 25
    The hospital identifies risks for the transmission and acquisition of infectious agents
        throughout the hospital 26
    The risk analysis is formally reviewed at least annually and whenever significant changes occur ...27
    Surveillance activities are used to identify infection prevention and control risks 28

Contents

Chapter Three: Priorities and goals for preventing transmission of HAIs 31
Priorities are established and goals related to preventing the acquisition and transmission
of potentially infectious agents are developed, based on the risks identified 32
Limiting unprotected exposure to pathogens throughout the hospital 32
Enhancing hand hygiene 32
This element of performance is currently in field review 33
Minimizing the risk of transmission of infections associated with the use of procedures,
medical equipment, and medical devices 33

Chapter Four: Strategies to achieve IC goals 35
Interventions are designed to incorporate relevant guidelines for infection prevention
and control activities 36
Interventions are implemented 38

Chapter Five: Effectiveness of IC interventions 53
The hospital formally evaluates and revises the goals and program (or portions of the program)
at least annually and whenever risks are significantly changed 53
The evaluation addresses changes in the scope of the IC program and changes in the results
of the IC program risk analysis 54
The evaluation addresses emerging and reemerging problems in the healthcare community
that potentially affect the hospital 54
The evaluation addresses the assessment of the success or failure of interventions
for preventing and controlling infection 54
The evaluation addresses responses to concerns raised by leadership and others
within the hospital 56
The evaluation addresses the evolution of relevant infection prevention and control guidelines
that are based on evidence or, in the absence of evidence, expert consensus 56

Chapter Six: Influx of infectious patients 57
The organization plans its response to an influx, or risk of an influx, of infectious patients 58
The organization has a plan for managing an influx of potentially infectious
patients/residents/clients over an extended period of time 58
The organization determines how it will keep abreast of current information about
the emergence of epidemics or new infections that may result in the organization
activating its response, determines how it disseminate critical information to staff
and other key practitioners, and identifies resources in the community 58

Chapter Seven: Effective management of the IC program 61

The hospital assigns responsibility for managing IC program activities to one or more individuals whose number, competency, and skill mix are determined by the goals and objectives of the IC activities 62

Qualifications of the individual(s) responsible for managing the IC program are determined by the risks entailed in the services provided, the hospital's patient population(s), and the complexity of the activities that will be carried out 66

This individual(s) coordinates all infection prevention and control within the hospital 66

This individual(s) facilitates ongoing monitoring of the effectiveness of prevention and/or control activities and interventions 67

Chapter Eight: Collaboration in implementing the IC program 69

Hospital leaders including medical staff, LIPs, and other direct and indirect patient care staff (including, when applicable, pharmacy, laboratory, administration, central supply/sterilization services, housekeeping, building maintenance/engineering, and food services) collaborate on an ongoing basis with the qualified individual(s) managing the IC program 70

These representatives participate in the development of strategies for each component's/function's role in the IC program; assessment of the adequacy of the human, information, physical, and financial resources allocated to support infection prevention and control activities; assessment of the overall failure or success of key processes for preventing and controlling infection; review and revision of the IC program as warranted to improve outcomes 70

Chapter Nine: Adequate resources for the IC program 73

Leaders review on an ongoing basis (but no less frequently than annually) the effectiveness of the hospital's infection prevention and control activities and report their findings to the integrated patient safety program 74

Adequate systems to access information are provided to support infection prevention and control activities 74

When applicable, adequate laboratory support is provided to support infection prevention and control activities 74

Adequate equipment and supplies are provided to support infection prevention and control activities 75

Introduction to chapters 10 and 11 77

Chapter 10: Hand-hygiene safety goal 79

Safety Goal #7: Reduce the risk of healthcare-acquired infections. 79

Goal #7a: Comply with current CDC hand-hygiene guidelines 79

CONTENTS

Chapter 11: Sentinel event safety goal 91
Safety Goal #7: Reduce the risk of healthcare-acquired infections 91
Safety goal #7b: Manage as sentinel events all identified cases of unanticipated death
or major permanent loss of function associated with a healthcare-associated infection 91

Chapter 12: Other standards related to IC 103
Human resources 103
Leadership 104
Environment of care 104
Performance improvement 105

Chapter 13: Designing a plan for JCAHO survey readiness 115
Mock survey 115

Chapter 14: Scoring guidelines: How to make sure you're successful 123
Designing a strategy to ensure a compliant score 123
Scoring categories 124
Compliance with the standard 127

Using the files on your Infection Control Compliance Guide: Understanding the JCAHO's 2005 Standards CD-ROM 130

About the author

Gail Bennett, RN, MSN, CIC

Gail Bennett, RN, MSN, CIC, has been involved in infection control (IC) for 26 years. She is executive director of Georgia-based ICP Associates, LLC, serves as a consultant to hospitals, nursing homes, and industry professionals, and provides presentations for professional associations. She also consults with IC programs in 259 healthcare facilities through their corporate offices.

Bennett has served on the Association for Professionals in Infection Control and Epidemiology (APIC) national board of directors, on the APIC-Atlanta board of directors, and on the board of directors and as treasurer for the national Center for Clinical Epidemiology. She currently serves on the board of directors of the Georgia Infection Control Network.

She has authored numerous chapters for APIC on IC and consulting. She is also author of *Getting Started: A Handbook for Nurse Consultants*, IC manuals for hospitals and nursing homes, and several journals. In addition, Bennett co-authored HCPro's 2004 book, *Infection Control Manual for Hospitals*.

Her consulting experience has covered the topics of IC, performance improvement, JCAHO survey preparation, and management.

She started and coordinates ICP Associates' annual three-day program "Surveillance, Prevention and Control of Healthcare-Associated Infections," which is held in Atlanta. In addition, she started and presents two-day training programs for IC professionals in long-term care in multiple states. She also serves as a motivational and educational speaker in numerous states each year.

Find out more about Bennett at her Web site, *www.icpassociates.com*.

How to use this book

This book helps you get ready for the infection control (IC) component of the Joint Commission on Accreditation of Healthcare Organizations (JCAHO) survey. Each chapter includes an overview of the pertinent IC standards; ideas for demonstrating compliance with each element of performance; and forms, policies, and templates.

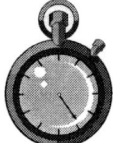 Look for this icon, which highlights policies and procedures throughout the book that will save you time in preparing for survey.

I encourage you to customize the material in this book to fit the needs of your facility. The accompanying CD-ROM contains many of the book's forms, policies, and templates for you to customize.

Chapters one through six pertain to the IC program and its components. Chapters seven through 14 deal with the structure and resources for the IC program.

Chapter summaries

Chapter 1: This chapter reviews the importance of an organization-wide IC program. It includes a template for establishing an IC plan and focuses on "authority" to take actions, communication, reporting of infections, investigation of outbreaks, and development of a written IC plan.

Chapter 2: This chapter focuses on completion of a risk analysis as part of the written IC plan.

Chapter 3: This chapter guides you in using the risk analysis to establish priorities and to set goals for preventing infections.

Chapter 4: This chapter reviews the strategies you need to meet your IC goals. It includes information on the use of appropriate national guidelines for prevention and control, hand hygiene, methods of reducing risk, appropriate precautions to take, and screening for exposure/immunity to infectious diseases.

Chapter 5: This chapter provides information on evaluating the effectiveness of IC interventions and, if needed, methods for redesigning and putting in place new interventions.

Chapter 6: This chapter prepares you to comply with the new standard that requires planning your facility's response to an influx or risk of influx of infectious patients, determining methods of obtaining current information, disseminating information, and identifying community resources.

Chapter 7: This chapter reviews the standard that requires effective management of your program. It addresses the qualifications and competencies of individuals responsible for managing the IC program. It also provides an IC competency assessment for use as either a self-assessment or as your facility's formal competency assessment for the infection control professional (ICP).

Chapter 8: This chapter addresses the need for hospital leaders to work together to establish and evaluate their IC programs.

Chapter 9: This chapter discusses how leaders allocate adequate resources for the IC program. It also provides a checklist you can use to evaluate whether your IC program has adequate resources available.

Chapter 10: This chapter reviews the JCAHO National Patient Safety Goal #7a, which requires compliance with current Centers for Disease Control and Prevention hand-hygiene guidelines.

Chapter 11: This chapter addresses the controversial subject of healthcare-associated infections (HAI) as sentinel events. It provides the tools to determine whether an HAI qualifies as a sentinel event.

Chapter 12: This chapter includes information on standards that may impact IC but are found outside the IC function.

Chapter 13: This chapter assists you in designing a plan for JCAHO survey readiness. It includes a template of the standards and elements of performance that may be used in a mock survey. It also provides tips on general survey preparation and interactions with surveyors.

Chapter 14: This chapter provides an overview of the scoring guidelines. It includes a review of the compliance track records needed to achieve the best scores as well as other factors that may impact the scores.

Introduction

The discipline of infection control (IC) and epidemiology in the United States has evolved dramatically over the past three decades. The Joint Commission on Accreditation of Healthcare Organizations (JCAHO) is credited with acknowledging IC as an important field in the 1970s, when it first included IC in its standards. This JCAHO action provided the thrust needed to propel this discipline into most healthcare arenas. However, other important issues have moved this field into prominence as well.

Presenting another of these issues, the Centers for Disease Control and Prevention (CDC) estimates that, annually, approximately two million patients admitted to acute-care hospitals in the United States acquire infections unrelated to the condition that required hospitalization.[1] These infections cause approximately 90,000 deaths and increase patient costs by $4.5 to $5.7 billion dollars each year.[2] In addition, emerging pathogens/infectious diseases such as monkey pox, mad cow disease, and avian influenza; the challenges of preventing transmission of multi-drug resistant organisms; and the threat of bioterrorism helped bring IC to critical importance.

Overview of 2005 standards

In keeping with its long-term role as an activist for IC, the JCHAO provides new challenges for IC programs in its 2005 standards. First, it emphasizes that hospitals should use responsive, and collaborative processes to develop, put into practice, and evaluate their IC programs.

It also emphasizes the need to involve organization leaders in supporting and evaluating those programs. The revised standards also require a written IC plan. The plan must include prioritized risks; program goals; strategies to minimize, reduce, or eliminate the risks; and a description of how to evaluate the strategies. It should become a dynamic document that reflects the evaluation and redesign of the program required under the standards.

A major addition to the standards is standard IC.6.10, which directs organizations to prepare, as part of emergency management activities, how they would respond to an influx or risk of an influx of infectious patients. Although emergency management plans generally address receiving patients during an emergency or disaster, this standard requires specific plans for receiving patients with infections and providing care to them over an extended period of time.

A continuation from previous JCAHO requirements is safety goal #7, which requires compliance with current CDC hand-hygiene guidelines. It also requires that facilities manage as sentinel events all identified cases of unanticipated death or major permanent loss of function in connection with a healthcare-associated infection (HAI). IC programs have struggled with managing HAIs as sentinel events, and over time, they have developed processes to identify them, follow their facility's reporting procedure, and complete a root-cause analysis effectively.

Compliance and beyond

The 2005 JCAHO standards for IC are challenging, but IC programs have excelled for decades at facing and conquering new challenges. The following is a list of specific steps to help you become compliant with the standards:

1. Study the standards, their rationale, and their elements of performance.
2. Conduct a self-assessment of current compliance.
3. Develop a detailed to-do list to maintain compliance with all standards (see Figure I.1 at the end of this chapter for an example).
4. Put in place the follow-up actions identified in the to-do list.
5. Reassess compliance with the standards.
6. Revise the to-do list for any areas that still need improvement.
7. Put into practice the additional actions noted in the to-do list.
8. Initiate a mock survey of the IC program and review compliance with the standards. Knowledgeable, objective reviewers should conduct the mock survey (see Figure 13.1 in Chapter 13 for a sample checklist to use in a mock survey).
9. Take action related to any areas needing improvement the mock survey identifies.
10. Share your excellent program with the JCAHO surveyors.

It is my hope that this book will provide you with information and ideas to help you accomplish your goals of developing an excellent IC program and completing a successful JCAHO survey.

Figure I.1 — Compliance To-Do List

IC Standard	Met?		If not met	
	Yes	No	Responsible person	Date project to be in compliance
IC 1.10 EP5: Is there a system in place to report identified infections to the receiving organization when a patient was transferred and the presence of an HAI was not known at the time of transfer?	☐	☐	ICP in collaboration with the clinical director	
IC 5.10 EP5: Does the infection control plan clearly evaluate the success or failure of interventions for preventing and controlling infections?	☐	☐	IC Staff in collaboration with the Performance Improvement Coordinator	
IC 6.10: Does the emergency management plan clearly address plans for responding to an influx of potentially infectious patients?	☐	☐	ICP in collaboration with the Safety Director	
IC 7.10 EP2: Does the personnel file(s) of the ICP(s) clearly document qualifications for managing the IC program?	☐	☐	IC staff and Human Resources Director	
IC 9.10 EP1: Is there a system in place to clearly document at least an annual review of the IC program activities by the leaders?	☐	☐	IC staff IC Supervisor Leadership representative	

References

1. CDC, "Monitoring hospital-acquired infections to promote patient safety—United States, 1990-1999. MMWR 49, no. 8 (March 3, 2000): 149–153.

2. CDC, "Public health focus: surveillance, prevention and control of nosocomial infections," MMWR 41, no. 92 (October 23, 1992): 783–7.

CHAPTER ONE

Organization-wide IC program

> **Review of the standard:**
>
> **IC.1.10** The risk of development of a healthcare-associated infection (HAI) is minimized through an organization-wide infection control (IC) program.

This chapter reviews the importance of an organization-wide IC program and focuses on authority for taking actions within the program, communication, reporting of infections, investigation of outbreaks, and development of a written IC plan. It includes a template for establishing an IC plan.

How to survey the standard:
- Interview IC staff
- Interview department managers
- Interview leadership

Documents that may be requested or reviewed:
- Organization-wide IC policies and procedures
- Infection reporting records
- Written IC plan
- Outbreak investigation documentation

CHAPTER ONE

Elements of performance for IC.1.10

> **1. An organization-wide IC program is implemented.**

IC must involve every aspect of the healthcare organization. Organization-wide involvement will be reflected in minutes of the IC committee, department-specific policies and procedures, the written IC plan, feedback provided to staff related to IC, and inservice and educational programs related to IC.

Department managers and organizational leaders should know the IC program well and be able to discuss it with the JCAHO surveyor. Staff level personnel should understand IC as it relates to their responsibilities.

> **2. Individuals and/or positions with the authority to take steps to prevent or control the acquisition and transmission of infectious agents are identified.**

Identify one person to handle the infection control professional's (ICP) duties and provide that person with an appropriate job description, which should outline aspects of the ICP's authority (see Figure 1.1 on page 3 for a sample job description for an ICP).

A hospital authority statement will further define the power of other specific staff to take actions in emergency situations (see Figure 1.2 on page 6 for a sample authority statement). Facility leaders must authorize the use of the authority statement.

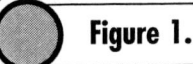

ICP Job Description

POSITION TITLE: Infection Control Professional

REPORTS TO: Administration

JOB SUMMARY:

Evaluates quality of patient care and patient outcomes as they relate to healthcare-associated infections; collects, prepares and analyzes healthcare-associated infection data; presents infection data and makes recommendations for actions; monitors employee compliance in use of barriers and infection prevention measures; prepares and presents educational offerings for the staff; serves as a resource to all departments and personnel; implements programs to protect the healthcare workers, visitors, and others in the healthcare environment; sets and recommends policies and procedures to prevent adverse events; provides internal and external reporting of information and data; promotes compliance with regulations, guidelines, and accreditation requirements.

QUALIFICATIONS:
- Holds a current state license as an LPN, RN, or medical technologist or has equivalent healthcare experience.
- Completion of a basic training program for infection control.
- Certification in Infection Control is desired.
- Ability to develop policies and procedures.
- Ability to teach and evaluate clinical performance.

DUTIES AND RESPONSIBILITIES:
1. Does on-going monitoring of healthcare-associated infections.
2. Assesses infection control problems and makes recommendations for corrective action.
3. Prepares the agenda for the Infection Control Committee.
4. Monitors infection control practices and employee compliance.
5. Serves as a resource for all departments and personnel.
6. Initiates and revises infection control policies and procedures.
7. Conducts outbreak investigation and initiates control measures.
8. Reports communicable diseases to the state as required by law.
9. Provides educational offerings for orientation and on-going inservices.
10. Consults with department heads and physicians as needed to improve care.
11. Initiates follow-up on employee/patient exposures to communicable diseases.
12. Participates in performance improvement activities.
13. Participates in short and long range planning for the infection control department.
14. Performs other duties as directed.

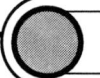

Figure 1.1 ICP Job Description (cont.)

PHYSICAL AND SENSORY REQUIREMENTS:
(With or without the Aid of Mechanical Devices)
- Must be able to move intermittently throughout the work day.
- Must be able to speak and write the English language in an understandable manner.
- Must be able to cope with the mental and emotional stress of the position.
- Must possess sight/hearing senses or use prosthetics that will enable these senses to function adequately so that the requirements of the position can be fully met.
- Must function independently, have flexibility, personal integrity, and the ability to work effectively with residents, personnel, and support agencies.
- Must meet the general health requirements set forth by the policies of this facility, which include a medical and physical examination.
- Must be able to push, pull, move, and/or lift a minimum of ___ pounds to a minimum height of ___ feet and able to push, pull, move, and/or carry such weight a minimum distance of ___ feet.
- May be necessary to assist in the evacuation of patients during emergency situations.

Acknowledgment

I have read this job description and fully understand the requirements set forth therein. I hereby accept the position of **Infection Control Professional** and agree to perform the identified essential functions in a safe manner and in accordance with the facility's established procedures. I understand that as a result of my employment, I may be exposed to blood, body fluids, infectious diseases, air contaminants (including tobacco smoke), and hazardous chemicals and that the facility will provide to me instructions on how to prevent and control such exposures. I further understand that I may also be exposed to the **Hepatitis B Virus** and that the facility will make available to me, free of charge, the hepatitis B immunization.

I understand that my employment is at-will, and thereby understand that my employment may be terminated at-will either by the facility or myself, and that such termination can be made with or without notice.

_____   _____
Date   Signature–Infection Control Professional

_____   _____
Date   Signature–Supervisor

> **3. All applicable organization components and functions are integrated into the IC program.**

Each facility determines which components and functions to integrate into the IC program. Facilities often integrate all clinical departments and services into the IC program, as well as multiple nonclinical departments such as environmental services, laundry services, maintenance, and safety and emergency management.

> **4. Systems are in place to communicate with licensed independent practitioners (LIP), staff, students/trainees, volunteers, and, as appropriate, visitors and patients about infection prevention and control issues, including their responsibilities in preventing the spread of infection within the hospital.**

Start the communication process by orienting LIPs, staff, students, trainees, and volunteers. Make the orientation specific to each group's department, service, and set of responsibilities. Communication should be ongoing, depending on the needs of each group.

Communication with visitors about infection prevention and control generally occurs at the unit level and may include verbal communication, use of instructional brochures/pamphlets, and posted notices (e.g., a notice entitled "Influenza Season").

Communication with patients generally involves education relating to infectious diseases, risks of procedures, and post-discharge instructions. Consider using closed-circuit television, pamphlets, and other written methods.

> **5. The hospital has systems for reporting identified infections to the following:**

- **The appropriate staff within the hospital**
  Establish methods for reporting infection information to appropriate staff based on their need to know. Such methods include verbal presentations, videos, private bulletin boards, and written information. Be aware of issues relating to confidentiality of the data.

- **Federal, state and local public health authorities in accordance with law and regulation**
  The IC program should be aware of external reporting requirements—such as from federal, state, and local public health agencies—and act accordingly.

CHAPTER ONE

- **Accrediting bodies**
  A facility might report an infection to the JCAHO if it is an HAI that qualifies as a sentinel event. In such a case, follow your facility's policies for sentinel event reporting (see Chapter 11 for information on infections as sentinel events).

- **The referring or receiving organization when a patient was transferred or referred and the presence of an HAI was not known at the time of referral.**
  There should be appropriate communication among healthcare organizations relating to HAIs (see Figure 1.3 for examples of instances when communication between facilities may be needed).

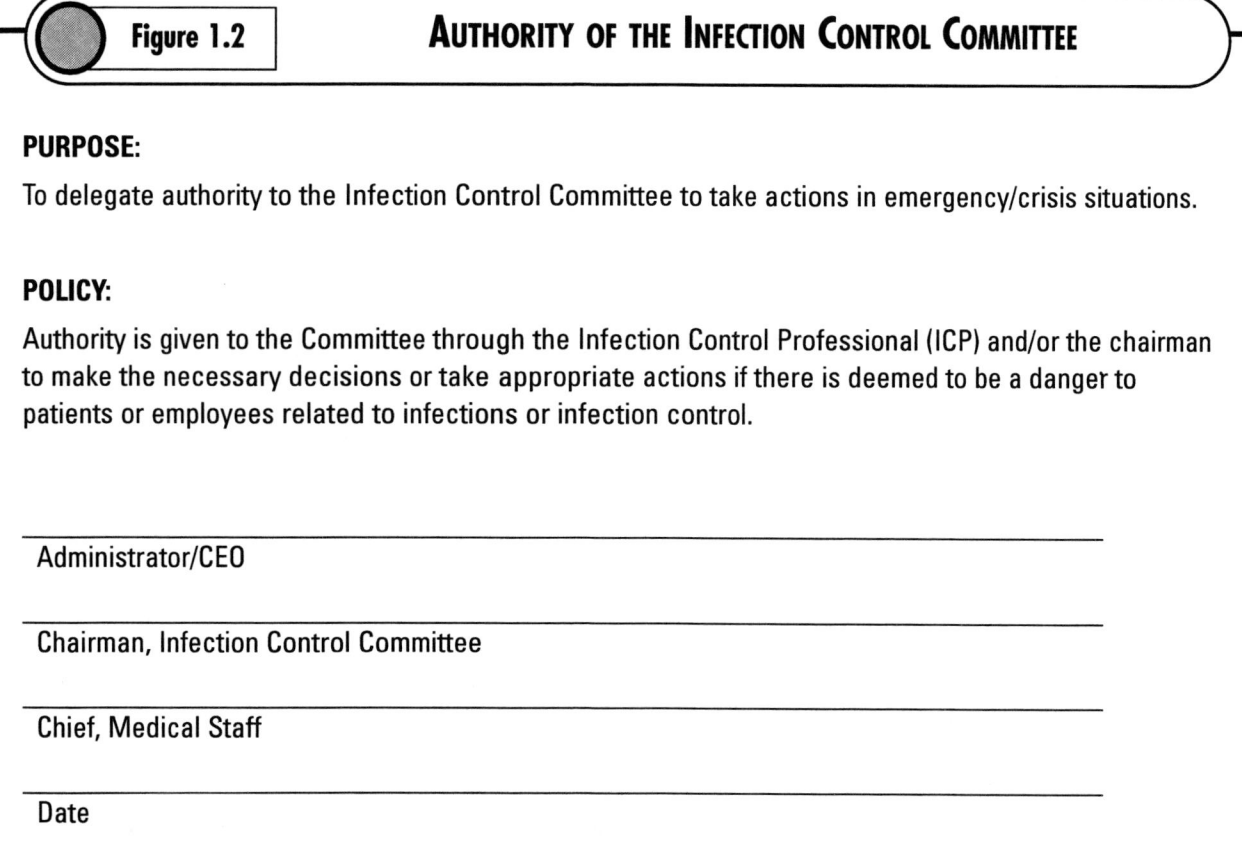

Figure 1.2 — AUTHORITY OF THE INFECTION CONTROL COMMITTEE

PURPOSE:
To delegate authority to the Infection Control Committee to take actions in emergency/crisis situations.

POLICY:
Authority is given to the Committee through the Infection Control Professional (ICP) and/or the chairman to make the necessary decisions or take appropriate actions if there is deemed to be a danger to patients or employees related to infections or infection control.

_____
Administrator/CEO

_____
Chairman, Infection Control Committee

_____
Chief, Medical Staff

_____
Date

Figure 1.3 — Communication Guide

Receiving organization communicating to referring organization	1. After admission by receiving organization, it is determined that the patient had a communicable disease, e.g., TB, that was not known during treatment by the referring organization. 2. The receiving organization determines that there is a surgical site infection within the first 30 days following surgery at the referring organization.
Referring organization communicating to the receiving organization	1. The referring organization notifies the receiving organization that cultures have been completed showing the presence of multi-drug resistant organisms. 2. After transfer to the receiving organization, the referring organization receives a culture report showing Mycobacterium tuberculosis.

6. Systems for investigating outbreaks of infectious diseases are in place.

Establish a process for timely detection/recognition of a potential outbreak. Once you detect an outbreak, use a systematic process for investigating it. Use the 10 specific steps of an outbreak investigation published by a variety of healthcare sources to conduct and report outbreaks (see Figure 1.4 on page 8 for a sample outbreak investigation policy and Figure 1.5 on page 10 for a sample form for conducting and documenting an outbreak. The form incorporates the 10 steps mentioned previously.)

Make policies and procedures relating to IC available to all your departments. In addition, make policies and procedures that are specific to the IC department available for use within the department and for review by surveyors (see Figure 1.6 on page 14 for a sample of a hospital IC manual's table of contents).

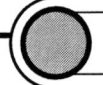

Figure 1.4 — **OUTBREAK INVESTIGATION**

DEFINITION

An outbreak is defined as two (2) or more cases over the usual (endemic) number of cases of healthcare-associated infections, usually produced by the same organism. The time period will vary according to the infection.

RECOGNITION AND NOTIFICATION

Any hospital personnel recognizing a possible epidemic will immediately report this to the Infection Control Department through which the Hospital Epidemiologist will be notified.

In the absence of the Hospital Epidemiologist, the Director of Infection Control, Infection Control Professional(s) (ICPs), or Microbiologist will be notified and temporarily substitute for the Hospital Epidemiologist in the following procedures:

PRELIMINARY INVESTIGATION

The Hospital Epidemiologist, or his/her designee, is designated as the Investigation Coordinator. He/she will review the charts of the involved patients and determine that an epidemic exists. The Investigation Coordinator, Microbiologist, ICP and Director of Nursing of the involved clinical area(s) will immediately confer and prepare a preliminary plan of investigation including the following:

A working definition of a case will be developed:
- The presumptive hypotheses for the mode of transmission of the organism and other circumstances will be developed. Procedures for testing the hypotheses will be outlined.

The Infection Control Department will gather and compile data related to the infection(s) as follows:
- Conduct case finding (review ongoing surveillance charts of other patients at risk and microbiology reports) to determine if there have been other cases of the infection
- Evaluate previous hospital experience with the infection
- Prepare a line listing of cases to include: hospital identification number, location in hospital, date of admission, date of infection onset, site culture results, medical service and attending physician
- Plot number of cases by date of onset (epidemic curve)
- Review patient charts of cases and interview involved hospital personnel for various factors that conceivably may have played a role in transmission of an infection, e.g., geographic locations of patients, specific personnel having contact with patients, medications, and treatments administered, etc.
- Review various infection control techniques (handwashing, sterile techniques, etc.) as actually practiced in the involved areas of the hospital
- Maintain surveillance for occurrence of any further infections

The Microbiologist will:
- Determine that all isolates of the involved organism(s) are saved for further study (e.g., biotyping, antimicrobial sensitivity patterns, phage typing, serotyping, etc.) as deemed appropriate. Subcultures are

Figure 1.4 — OUTBREAK INVESTIGATION (CONT.)

prepared for possible shipment to a reference laboratory.
- Determine what environmental and/or personnel cultures are to be taken by whom and by what technique.
- Determine what patient care items suspected of being possible sources of infection may need to be impounded or quarantined.

COMMUNICATIONS

The Hospital Epidemiologist will ensure that the following other individuals are notified concurrently with the preliminary investigation and advised at reasonable intervals of the progress of the investigation: attending physicians, the department chairman of the medical services involved, and the hospital administrator.

IMMEDIATE CONTROL

Reasonable immediate control measures are determined by the Hospital Epidemiologist or designee and put into effect on his/her authority in an attempt to halt the spread of infection. Such measures might include but are not limited to: isolation, suspension of certain elective procedures, removal of common suspected sources of personnel from patient contact, or immediate inservice training in certain infection control techniques.

PUBLIC INFORMATION

Any questions from the community, uninvolved hospital personnel, or news media are directed to the hospital administrator who will act as public information coordinator.

ANALYSIS OF DATA

The data collected in the preliminary investigation are reviewed by the investigators to determine if a common source of infection, break in technique, etc., can be implicated as the cause of the epidemic. A preliminary written report will be prepared.

FURTHER INVESTIGATION

If the cause of the infection is not evident as a result of the above investigation, a more detailed case control study using statistical epidemiologic methods may be required. The Hospital Epidemiologist may elect to consult the state health department and the USPHS Centers for Disease Control and Prevention for assistance with further studies.

CONCLUSION OF INVESTIGATION

The investigation is continued at least as long as there are cases of the infection occurring above the endemic level.

A final written report of the investigation, outlining findings and recommendations, is prepared by the investigation coordinator and issued to the Infection Control Committee, others participating in the investigation, attending physician(s), department chairpersons of the medical service(s) involved, and the hospital administrator.

CHAPTER ONE

Figure 1.5 — **OUTBREAK INVESTIGATION FORM**

1. Verify the diagnosis; identify the agent.

Describe the initial magnitude of the problem and what symptoms got the facility's attention.

What diagnosis has been established?

What agent (bacterial, viral, other) has been identified? (Review microbiology/laboratory records to identify cluster or confirm increase of certain pathogens. Consult with staff to identify problem and monitor use of infection control procedures.)

Develop a case definition (specific criteria for a case).
Example: All patients who have had loose stools for >12 hours.

CASE DEFINITION:

2. Confirm that an outbreak exists.

Use your case definition to find all cases.

Based on your knowledge in #1, are the numbers of cases above what is endemic (usually seen) in the facility? If yes, consider that an outbreak exists.	☐ Yes	☐ No
Total number of cases so far:	DATE:	
Do you have an outbreak? If yes, proceed.	☐ Yes	☐ No

Infection Control Compliance Guide: Understanding the JCAHO's Standards

Figure 1.5 — OUTBREAK INVESTIGATION FORM (CONT.)

3. Search for additional cases.

Encourage immediate reporting of cases (laboratory, physicians, personnel).

Search for other cases by retrospective record review, lab reports, etc.

Total number of cases: _____   DATE:

4. Characterize the cases by person, place, time.

Person: (Patient characteristics - age, sex, disease, exposures, treatments)

Place: (Consider ward, hall, room, outside exposures. May use facility maps. Check and confirm status of air exchange, pattern of flow (positive/negative) and environment as they relate to outbreak.)

Time: What is the period of the outbreak? What is the probable source of exposure?

Record dates of onset and draw an epidemic curve.

5. Form a tentative hypothesis (best guess at the time).

Review data to determine common host factors and exposures. Develop a best guess on the:

Reservoir

Source

Mode of transmission

Figure 1.5 — Outbreak Investigation Form (cont.)

6. Institute preliminary control measures.

Initiate control measures based on what you know (handwashing, isolation, cohorting, etc.). Determine if you need outside assistance.

Control measures:	
Date implemented:	
Assistance needed? ☐ Yes ☐ No	

7. Test the hypothesis.

Many hospital problems never reach this stage. It may end without intervention or simple control measures may cause the problem to cease.

Special epidemiologic studies may be needed and we may need to seek help.

8. Refine the control measures.

Additional measures, if needed:

ADDED

9. Monitor and evaluate the control measures

Are control measures being used appropriately?	☐ Yes ☐ No
If no, ensure compliance.	
Evaluate control measures. Did cases cease?	☐ Yes ☐ No
If no, consider additional actions.	

10. Prepare and disseminate a final report.

This form in a completed state may serve as the final report. Make the report as detailed as possible.

Date of final report:	
Reported to:	
Reported by:	

ORGANIZATION-WIDE IC PROGRAM

> **7. Applicable policies and procedures are in place throughout the hospital.**

Make policies and procedures relating to IC available to all your departments. In addition, make policies and procedures that are specific to the IC department available for use within the department and for review by surveyors (see Figure 1.6 at the end of this chapter for a sample of a hospital IC manual's table of contents).

> **8. Not Applicable.**

> **9. The hospital has a written IC plan that includes the following:**

- A description of prioritized risks
- A statement of the IC program's goals
- A description of the hospital's strategies to minimize, reduce, or eliminate the prioritized risks
- A description of how the strategies will be evaluated

The written IC plan should be a comprehensive, dynamic document that reflects the assessment of infection risks in the facility. It requires the following:
- An assessment of the geographic location and community environment
- The services provided
- Analysis of the hospital's infection data
- Care, treatment, and services provided by the facility

Once the risk assessment is complete, determine your program's goals and priorities, develop strategies, and determine which methods you'll use to evaluate the strategies (see Figure 1.7 on page 18 for an IC plan checklist). Review the IC plan at least annually and as needed due to changing circumstances.

Chapters two, three, four, and five of this book detail elements of the IC plan.

Figure 1.6 — Hospital Infection Control Manual Table of Contents

MANUAL APPROVAL FORM

INFECTION CONTROL PROGRAM: SECTION 1   **PAGE**

    Overview 1
    Plan of Surveillance, Prevention and Control 3
    Infection control practitioner job description 4
    Infection control committee 6
    Authority statement 7
    Sample minutes form 8

SURVEILLANCE OF INFECTIONS: SECTION 2

    Surveillance policy 1
    CDC Definitions of Nosocomial Infections 2
    Reportable diseases 20
    Infection Line Listing 21
    Infection Worksheet By Site And Organism 22
    Surgical Site Infections Worksheet By Surgical Service 23
    Outbreak Investigation 24
    Outbreak investigation form 27

INFECTION CONTROL EDUCATION: SECTION 3

    Orientation and inservice 1
    Orientation outline 2
    OSHA bloodborne pathogens outline 4
    TB employee training outline 7

ISOLATION FOR COMMUNICABLE DISEASES: SECTION 4

    Standard precautions 1
    Contact precautions 3
    Droplet precautions 5
    Airborne Precautions 6
    Respiratory Protection Program for Airborne Infectious Diseases 8
    Tasks/Operations Requiring Respiratory Protection 12
    Respiratory Protection Exposure Determination
    For Biological Agents (TB and Smallpox) 13
    Epidemiologically Significant Organisms 14
    Compliance monitoring 16
    Staff self-evaluation 17
    Monitoring compliance with practices 18
    Using gloves 19
    Appendix A: CDC Guidelines: Type and Duration of Precautions
    Needed for Selected Infections and Conditions 21

EMPLOYEE HEALTH: SECTION 5

    Health Assessment/Evaluation 1
    Annual TB assessment (For use with staff who are PPD Positive) 2
    Reporting employee infections 3
    Employee infection record 4

Figure 1.6 — HOSPITAL INFECTION CONTROL MANUAL TABLE OF CONTENTS (CONT.)

Summary of Important Recommendations And Work Restrictions For
    Personnel With Infectious Diseases 5
Table – Recommendations And Work Restrictions For Personnel With Infectious Diseases 6
Criteria for determining exposure to communicable diseases 10
Management of accidental exposure to communicable diseases 12
Influenza vaccine and Healthcare Personnel 15
Influenza Vaccine Informed Consent Form 16
Hepatitis B Immunization Program 17
Hepatitis B Vaccine Information 18
Hepatitis B Vaccine Consent/Declination Form 19
Tuberculosis Screening For Employees 20
Bloodborne Pathogens 24
Post-Exposure Evaluation And Follow-Up 26
Healthcare Professional's Written Opinion 29
Hepatitis B Exposure Prophylaxis 30
Potential HIV Exposure 31
Consent Form For HIV Testing 32
Vaccine Recommendations 33
Pregnant Personnel 34
Frequently Asked Questions: TB 35

GENERAL PATIENT CARE POLICIES: SECTION 6
    Cleaning, Disinfection And Sterilization 1
    Management of Positive Biological Indicator In A Steam Sterilizer 2
    Table: Comparisons & Definitions of Sterilization And Disinfection 3
    Approved Sterilizing, Disinfecting and Hand Hygiene Agents 5
    Environmental Sampling 6
    Hand Hygiene 7
    Handling and/or Disposing of Used Needles 9
    Personal Hygiene 10
    Intravenous Therapy 11
    Table: Catheters used for Venous and arterial access 14
    Respiratory Care 15
    Reprocessing of Single-Use Medical Devices By Hospitals 17
    Animals in the Hospital 18
    Patient Immunizations 20
    Collection of Specimens 21
    Supply Check 22
    Use of Thermometers 23
    Management of Clean Equipment 24
    Endoscopes 25
    Feeding Syringes 27
    Nasogastric/Gastronomy Tube Feeding 28
    Total Parenteral Nutrition 29
    Urinary Catheters 30
    Visitors 31
    Infectious Waste Management 32
    Prevention of Wound Infections 34
    Wound Care Procedure For Major Wounds 35

Figure 1.6 — Hospital Infection Control Manual Table of Contents (cont.)

    Staple Removal 37
    Management of Pressure Ulcers 38
    Traffic Control 39

DEPARTMENT POLICIES: SECTION 7
    Central Sterile Processing 1
    Dietary Services 4
    Vending Room (Canteen) 9
    Laboratory 10
    Laundry 13
    Pharmacy 15
    Physical Therapy 18
    Respiratory Therapy 21
    Radiology And Nuclear Medicine 22
    Surgical Services 23

OSHA BLOODBORNE PATHOGENS EXPOSURE CONTROL PLAN: SECTION 8
    Exposure control plan 1
    Purpose 1
    Policy 1
    Program Administration 2
    Employee exposure determination 2
    Methods of Implementation and Control 3
    Standard Precautions 3
    Exposure Control Plan 3
    Engineering Controls and Work Practices 3
    Personal Protective Equipment 4
    Housekeeping 5
    Laundry 5
    Labels 6
    Hepatitis B Vaccination 6
    Post-Exposure Evaluation and Follow-up 6
    Administration of Post-Exposure Evaluation and Follow-up 7
    Procedures for Evaluating the Circumstances Surrounding an Exposure Incident 7
    Employee Training 8
    Recordkeeping 8
    Training Records 8
    Medical Records 9
    OSHA Recordkeeping 9
    Sharps Injury Log 9
    Table: Sample Sharps Injury Log 10
    Hepatitis B Vaccine Declination (Mandatory Wording) 11
    Form for employee input – engineering and work practice controls 12

TUBERCULOSIS CONTROL PLAN: SECTION 9
    Administrative Controls 1
    Assignment of Responsibility 1
    Risk Assessment 2

Figure 1.6 — HOSPITAL INFECTION CONTROL MANUAL TABLE OF CONTENTS (CONT.)

    Admissions 2
    Prospective Employees 3
    Annual Personnel Screening 3
    Exposure Incidents 3
    Documentation of Occupational Exposure 4
    Information And Training 4
    Engineering Controls 4
    Personal Protective Equipment 4
    TB Risk Assessment Form 6
    Elements of A TB Infection Control Program 7
    Employee TB Skin Testing Summary 10
    Annual Employee Tuberculosis Assessment 11

ENVIRONMENT OF CARE: SECTION 10
    Overview 1
    Construction and Renovation in the Healthcare Facility ... 2
    Housekeeping Services 5
    Ice Chests and Ice Machines 8
    Maintenance Department 9
    Maintenance Procedures in High Risk Units 11
    Pest Control 12

HEALTH INSURANCE PORTABILITY AND ACCOUNTABILITY ACT of 1996 (HIPAA): SECTION 11

BIOTERRORISM PLAN: SECTION 12
    Introduction 3
    General Categorical Recommendations for Any
    Suspected Bioterrorism Event 3
    Potential Agents 4
    Detection of Outbreaks caused by Agents of Bioterrorism ... 4
    Infection Control Practices for Patient Management ... 5
    Post Exposure Management 8
    Patient, Visitor, and Public Information 10
    Disease specific information
    Anthrax 11
    Botulism 16
    Plague 19
    Smallpox 23
    Reference List 27
    Federal Bureau of Investigation (FBI) Field Offices ... 28
    Public Health Offices - Contact Information 29
    Web sites and other Sources of Information 34

SUGGESTED REFERENCE BOOKS: SECTION 13

Source: HCPro, Infection Control Manual for Hospitals, 2004

Chapter One

Figure 1.7 — Infection Control Plan

This plan has been developed by the Infection Control Committee with input and collaboration from the following:
- Safety Committee
- Performance Improvement Committee
- Leadership including Department Managers
- Chief of Services

A risk assessment is a component of this plan. The plan and risk assessment are formally reviewed at lease annually and whenever significant changes occur in the elements that affect risk.

Risk Assessment

Date: _____

Factors	Characteristics that increase risks	Characteristics that decrease risks
Geographic location and community environment		
Care, treatment and services provided, e.g.: • Medical • Surgical • Pediatric • Emergency • Neonatal • Transplant		
Population characteristics		

Analysis of infection prevention and control data

	Problem-prone
High risk	

	Improvement needed
High Volume	

Figure 1.7 — Infection Control Plan (cont.)

Based on the risk assessment, the facility has identified the following risks and prioritized them in descending order:

Priority	Risk

Figure 1.7 — Infection Control Plan (cont.)

For each prioritized risk, identify goals, strategies, responsible person, time frame, and evaluation of effectiveness

RISKS	GOALS	STRATEGIES	IMPLEMENTATION		
			Responsible Persons	Timeframe	Method and Evaluation of Effectiveness

Infection Control Plan reviewed by:

_____ Date _____ Date

_____ Date _____ Date

_____ Date _____ Date

_____ Date _____ Date Leadership representative

_____ Date _____ Date Leadership representative

ORGANIZATION-WIDE IC PROGRAM

Figure 1.7 — **INFECTION CONTROL PLAN (CONT.)**

Based on the analysis of infection prevention and control data, complete the surveillance plan.

Important Aspects of Care	Indicators	Benchmarks	Data Source	Data Collector	Sample	Collected/ Tabulated/ Reported
SURVEILLANCE of Healthcare-Associated Infections, targeted to High-risk problem-prone infections	**EXAMPLE** Ventilator-related pneumonia	**EXAMPLE** To be established using P-charts	**EXAMPLE** Medical records, lab reports, staff clinical evaluations	**EXAMPLE** Infection Control Professional (ICP)	**EXAMPLE** 100% of ventilated patients in ICU	**EXAMPLE** Ongoing, Monthly/Quarterly

Infection Control Compliance Guide: Understanding the JCAHO's Standards

Introduction to chapters two, three, four, and five

The next four chapters address actions that will become part of the infection control (IC) plan. These actions include the following:

1. Identifying and prioritizing risks
2. Setting goals
3. Developing strategies
4. Evaluating the effectiveness of the strategies

The following schematic depicts each step of the process of developing and communicating the IC plan:

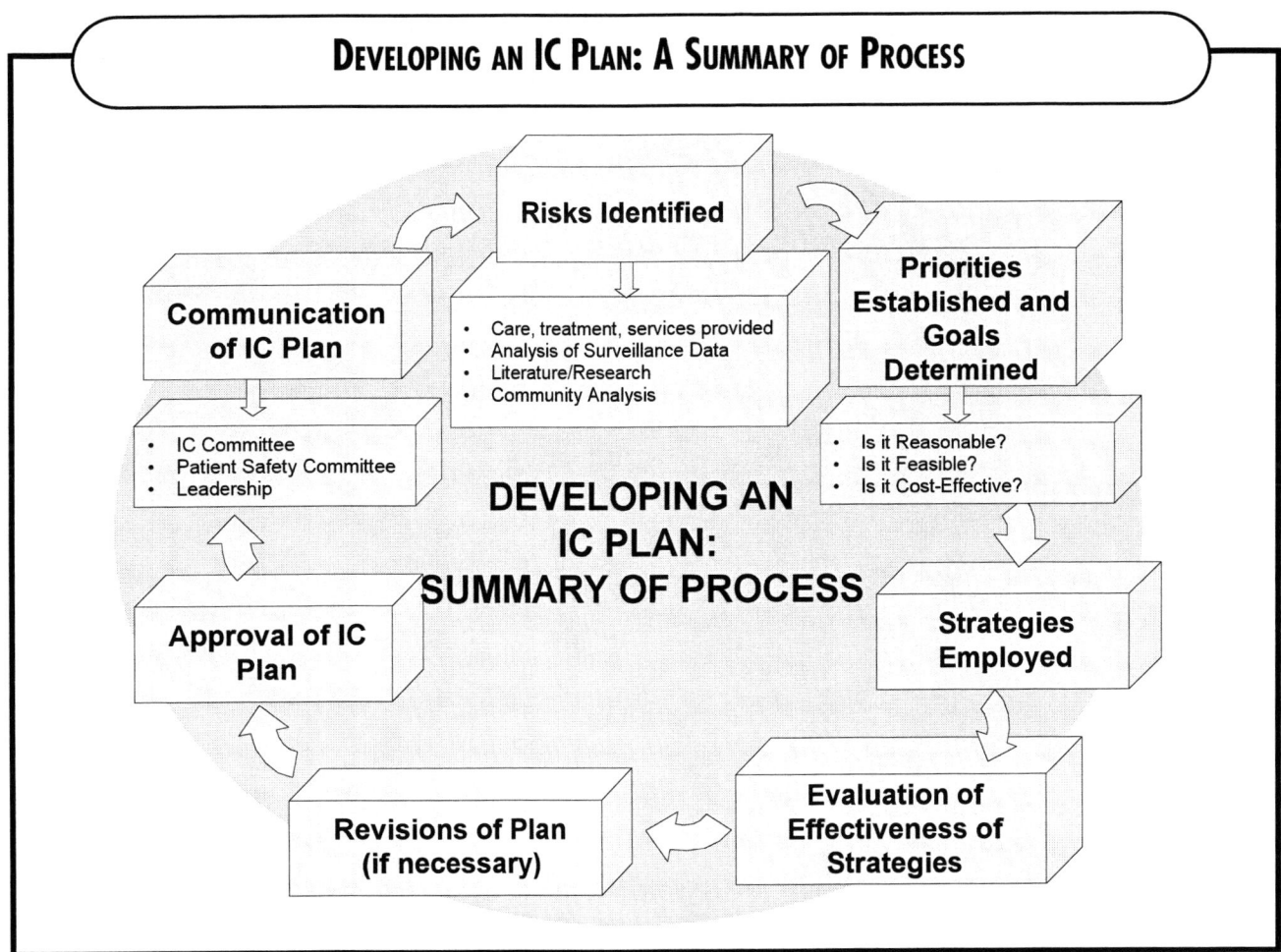

CHAPTER TWO

Risks for acquisition and transmission of infectious agents

Review of the standard:

IC.1.20 The infection control (IC) program identifies risks for the acquisition and transmission of infectious agents on an ongoing basis.

This chapter focuses on completing a risk analysis as part of the written IC plan.

How to survey the standard:
- Interview IC staff
- Interview department managers

Documents that may be requested or reviewed:
- Written IC plan/risk analysis
- Surveillance plan
- Surveillance data

CHAPTER TWO

Elements of Performance for IC.2.10

> 1. The hospital identifies risks for the transmission and acquisition of infectious agents throughout the hospital based on the following factors:

- **The geographic location and community environment of the hospital, services provided, and the characteristics of the population served**

  Each geographic area and community has unique issues relating to infectious diseases. For example, Hawaii has a high endemic rate of tuberculosis (TB), which a facility would need to consider when developing an IC plan. Some urban communities have large numbers of homeless people and therefore have special concerns relating to infectious diseases. Communities with elevated rates of illegal intravenous drug use may have high incidences of bloodborne pathogens, including human immunodeficiency virus (HIV), and other communities may have a high number of community-acquired methicillin-resistant *Staphylococcus aureus* (MRSA) cases.

  Each of these unique community characteristics affect development of your hospital IC plan. Some variations in the presence of infectious diseases may be well known in the healthcare community, but others may not. Therefore, regularly review the state's epidemiology reports of infectious diseases to help determine your geographic or community risk factors. The Centers for Disease Control and Prevention's (CDC) *Morbidity and Mortality Weekly Report* (MMWR) is another great resource for such information. Find the MMWR at www.cdc.gov/mmwr.

- **The results of the analysis of the hospital's infection prevention and control data**

  Many hospital IC programs excel at analyzing their infection prevention and control data. This analysis is critical to the design of the IC plan. Therefore, in assessing IC data, examine the following at four areas of concern:

- High-risk areas/issues

  Determine areas of high risk in your facility. Examples include
  — transplant services
  — TB unit
  — immunocompromised patients
  — burn unit
  — intensive care units
  — specific surgical procedures with high past infection rates

- High-volume infections or procedures

    The facility should consider what services are provided, infections are observed, or procedures are performed in high volume. Examples include
    — central lines
    — coronary artery bypass grafts (CABG)
    — TB cases
    — transplants
    — hemodialysis

- Problem-prone issues

    Each facility has a history of problem-prone issues relating to infections. These issues generally can be identified by reviewing past surveillance data and IC committee minutes. Once issues are identified, laboratory data can help assess pathogens of significance in the facility.

- Improvement needed

    Most healthcare facilities are acutely aware of IC issues that need improvement. IC and performance improvement committees generally maintain data in areas needing improvement, and if that information is not readily available, gather it by
    — reviewing surveillance data
    — reviewing committee minutes
    — reviewing survey reports
    — conducting interviews with department managers
    — reviewing compliance monitoring
    — reviewing the care, treatment, and services provided

The specific care, treatment, and services provided by the hospital will impact greatly the contents of the IC plan. The exercise of identifying high-risk, high-volume, problem-prone issues and areas of improvement will provide you with most of the information you need about care, treatment, and services provided in the hospital.

> **2. The risk analysis is formally reviewed at least annually and whenever significant changes occur in any of the above factors.**

CHAPTER TWO

Many hospitals conduct annual evaluations of their IC programs and the risk analysis could become part of such an annual evaluation. In addition to being updated during the annual evaluation, the risk analysis should be updated any time there are significant changes in the population served; in the hospital's infection prevention and control data; and in the care, treatment, and services provided.

> **3. Surveillance activities are used to identify infection prevention and control risks pertaining to the following:**

- **Patients**

    Patients have always been the primary focus of infection surveillance and will continue to be its core.

- **Licensed independent practitioners (LIP), staff, volunteers, and students/trainees**

    Infection monitoring also focuses on LIPs, staff, volunteers, and students/trainees. IC should work closely with occupational health to oversee
    — testing for immunity
    — immunizations
    — infection reporting
    — work restrictions for communicable diseases
    — exposure criteria and follow-up

- **Visitors**

    Visitors play a role in infection transmission and also have the potential to acquire infections in the hospital. Therefore, many hospitals provide educational material about infection prevention and control to patients, families, and visitors. This material may include disease-specific information, procedure-specific risk, and isolation information.

Figure 2.1 on page 29 provides a management matrix that may facilitate your thinking about prioritizing risks. It asks the following questions for each potential area of risk:

- What is the risk of a negative impact or outcome?
- What is the likelihood of the event occurring?

Figure 2.1 — Risk Assessment

Risk assessment

In this chart, plot the events with risk of negative impact (e.g. specific type of infection) against the likelihood that they will occur.

Likelihood of events occurring	Risk of negative impact or outcome		
	Low 1	Medium 2	High 3
Improbable 1	1	2	3
Unlikely 2	2	4	6
Likely 3	3	6	9
Very likely 4	4	8	12

Adapted from Heller, R., and Hindle, T., NY: DK Publishing, Inc., 1998

To score an event, multiply risks by likelihood of occurrence. Two examples have been done here.

Scoring rationale examples

Events of Low risk category (1) whose likelihood of occurrence was improbable were multiplied by 1, to give a score of 1 to that event. (1 x 1 = 1)

Events of High risk category (3) whose likelihood of occurrence was very likely were multiplied by 4, to give a score of 12 to that event. (3 x 4 = 12)

The higher the score, the higher the issue's priority will be.

CHAPTER THREE

Priorities and goals for preventing transmission of HAIs

> **Review of the standard:**
> **IC.3.10** Based on the risks, the hospital establishes priorities and sets goals for preventing the development of healthcare-associated infections within the hospital.

This chapter provides guidance on using the risk analysis to establish priorities and to set goals for preventing infections.

> **How to survey the standard:**
> - Interview IC staff
> - Observe IC practices
>
> **Documents that may be requested or reviewed:**
> - Written IC plan/priorities and goals
> - Policies and procedures

Once your risk analysis is complete, set goals for minimizing identified risks. For example, if the risk analysis shows that your community has a high rate of tuberculosis (TB)—and surveillance data and your facility's annual TB risk assessment confirm that the hospital patient population reflects the community population—set goals for preventing TB transmission in the hospital environment. Then develop additional goals for other risks you identify and prioritize them.

CHAPTER THREE

When writing goals, keep these important questions in mind:

- Is the goal reasonable? Does it accurately address the identified risk?
- Is the goal feasible? Can it be accomplished within the specific hospital environment?
- Is it cost-effective? If it is not cost-effective, do the benefits outweigh the costs?

The JCAHO requires several of the goals that are to become part of the IC plan, including limiting exposure; enhancing hand hygiene; and minimizing transmission associated with procedures, medical equipment, and medical devices.

Elements of performance for IC.3.10

> **1. Priorities are established and goals related to preventing the acquisition and transmission of potentially infectious agents are developed, based on the risks identified. These goals include, but are not limited to, the following:**

> **2. Limiting unprotected exposure to pathogens throughout the hospital**

Limiting unprotected exposure to pathogens has always been a primary goal of the IC program. Multiple IC policies/processes address methods of achieving this goal, such as the following:

- Isolation and barrier precautions
- Personal protective equipment
- Airflow patterns
- Sharps safety programs
- Hand hygiene
- Sterilization, disinfection, and sanitation
- Visitor policies

> **3. Enhancing hand hygiene**

Appropriate handwashing and hand hygiene are also long-standing priorities of IC programs. Hand hygiene in healthcare has the potential for great improvement since the 2002 publication of the CDC's *Guideline for Hand Hygiene in Health-care Settings*, which strongly supports alcohol handrub use, convenient locations for handrubs, and monitoring for compliance with hand-hygiene policies. See Chapter 10 of this book for more information on hand hygiene.

Priorities and goals for preventing transmission of HAIs

> **4. Note: This element of performance is currently in field review. It will be provided in a future update as soon as it has been approved. Please refer to *Joint Commission Perspectives* newsletter for more information about this standard.**

> **5. Minimizing the risk of transmission of infections associated with the use of procedures, medical equipment, and medical devices.**

This goal focuses on minimizing transmission of infections associated with the following:

- Procedures
- Medical equipment
- Medical devices

Generally, hospitals have detailed policies and procedures relating to infection prevention and control in each of these three areas. In addition, the risk analysis identifies the risks perceived to be associated with specific procedures, allowing you to set procedure-specific goals (e.g., a goal to decrease surgical-site infections related to joint replacements). Likewise, some medical equipment and medical devices may present a risk relating to infection transmission (e.g., dialysis equipment), so set goals specific to preventing infection relating to equipment/device use.

CHAPTER FOUR

Strategies to achieve IC goals

Review of the standard:
IC.4.10 Once the hospital has prioritized its goals, strategies must be implemented to achieve the goals.

This chapter reviews strategies needed to meet your infection control (IC) goals. It includes information on appropriate national guidelines for prevention and control, hand hygiene, methods of reducing risk, appropriate precautions, and screening for exposure/immunity to infectious diseases.

How to survey the standard:
- Interview IC staff
- Interview department managers

Documents that may be requested or reviewed:
- Written IC plan/strategies
- Policies and procedures
- Minutes of the IC committee

CHAPTER FOUR

Elements of performance for IC.4.10

> 1. **Interventions are designed to incorporate relevant guidelines for infection prevention and control activities.**

IC guidelines, as well as Occupational Safety and Health Administration (OSHA) regulations that impact IC, are constantly changing. Therefore, it is imperative that your IC program put mechanisms in place to inform you of pertinent changes and to ensure that IC interventions and activities reflect the most current recommendations and regulations.

A variety of sources have developed infection prevention and control guidelines. Many of these resources reflect nationally accepted standards of practice, so consider them when developing IC strategies.

The Centers for Disease Control and Prevention (CDC) provides the following guidelines pertinent to IC (not an all-inclusive list):

- *Guidelines for Preventing the Transmission of Mycobacterium tuberculosis in Health-Care Facilities*
- *Guideline for Prevention of Catheter-Associated Urinary Tract Infections*
- *Guidelines for Preventing Health-Care Associated Pneumonia*
- *Guidelines for Infection Control in Health-Care Personnel*
- *Guidelines for Prevention of Surgical Site Infection*
- *Guidelines for the Prevention of Intravascular Catheter-Related Infections*
- *Recommendations for Preventing the Spread of Vancomycin Resistance*
- *Guidelines for Infection Control in Dental Health-Care Settings*
- *Guidelines for Environmental Infection Control in Health-Care Facilities*

Find the CDC guidelines at *www.cdc.gov/ncidod/hip/guide/guide.htm*.

The Association for Professionals in Infection Control and Epidemiology (APIC) has developed guidelines, position papers, professional and practice standards that are of importance to IC including the following:

Guidelines:
- APIC Guideline for Infection Prevention and Control in Flexible Endoscopy
- APIC Guideline for Selection and Use of Disinfectants

- Multi-Society Guideline for Reprocessing Flexible Gastrointestinal Endoscopes
  Infection Control in Cystic Fibrosis

APIC professional and practice standards:
- APIC/CHICA-Canada Professional and Practice Standards Task Force

APIC position statements:
- "Responsibility for Interpretation of PPD Tuberculin Skin Test"
- "Release of Nosocomial Infection Data"
- "Infection Prevention and Control in the Long-Term Care Facility"
- "Improving Health Care Worker Influenza Immunization Rates"
- "Clean vs. Sterile: Management of Chronic Wounds"
- "Hepatitis C Exposure in the Health Care Setting"
- "Integrating Sentinel Event Analysis into Your Infection Control Practice"

Find the APIC guidelines at *www.apic.org* under "Practice Guidance."

The Society for Healthcare Epidemiologists of America (SHEA) also has IC guidelines, including the following:
- Multi-society guideline for reprocessing flexible gastrointestinal endoscopes
- SHEA guideline for preventing healthcare-associated transmission of multidrug-resistant strains of *Staphylococcus aureus* and *Enterococcus*
- Infection control recommendations for patients with cystic fibrosis, including microbiology, important pathogens, and infection control practices to prevent patient-to-patient transmission of infection
- Guidelines for the prevention of intravascular catheter-related infections.
- *Clostridium difficile* in long-term care facilities for the elderly
- Guideline for hand hygiene in healthcare settings: recommendations of the healthcare IC practices advisory committee and the HICPAC/SHEA/APIC/IDSA Hand Hygiene Task Force
- Requirements for infrastructure and essential activities of IC and epidemiology in hospitals: a consensus panel report
- Infection prevention and control in the long term-care facility
- How to select and interpret molecular strain typing methods for epidemiological studies of bacterial infections: a review for healthcare epidemiologists
- Management of healthcare workers infected with hepatitis B virus, hepatitis C virus, human immunodeficiency virus, or other bloodborne pathogens
- Guidelines for the prevention of antimicrobial resistance in hospitals
- Antimicrobial resistance in long-term-care facilities
- Antimicrobial use in long-term-care facilities

Chapter Four

- Clostridium difficile-associated diarrhea and colitis
- An approach to the evaluation of quality indicators of the outcome of care in hospitalized patients, with a focus on healthcare-associated infection indicators
- Medical waste

Additionally, SHEA makes available a variety of textbooks and journals that provide current IC information and standards of practice. Find the SHEA guidelines at *www.shea-online.org/publications/shea_position_papers.cfm*.

> **2. Interventions are implemented which include the following:**

a. An organization-wide hand-hygiene program that complies with current CDC hand-hygiene guidelines (National Patient Safety Goal #7, requirement 7a). See Chapter 10 for a discussion of this safety goal.

b. Methods to reduce the risks associated with procedures, medical equipment, and medical devices, including the following:
- **Appropriate storage, cleaning, disinfection, sterilization, and/or disposal of supplies and equipment**
- **Reuse of equipment designated by the manufacturer as disposable in a manner that is consistent with regulatory and professional standards**
- **The appropriate use of personal protective equipment**

Establish policies and procedures that address each of those three areas. Some resources that may help you to develop/revise these policies include

- storage, cleaning, disinfection, sterilization, and/or disposal of supplies and equipment
    - APIC Guideline on Sterilization
    - APIC Text of Infection Control and Epidemiology, Second Edition, 2005
    - See www.apic.org for further information

- reuse of equipment
    - See Figure 4.1 for the Food and Drug Administration (FDA) brochure titled "Reprocessing of Single-Use Medical Devices by Hospitals." Access it at *www.fda.gov/cdrh/reuse/trifold1.pdf*

STRATEGIES TO ACHIEVE IC GOALS

Figure 4.1 — **REPROCESSING OF SINGLE-USE MEDICAL DEVICES BY HOSPITALS**

Because insufficient data exist regarding the safety of reprocessing single-use devices (SUD), the U.S. Food and Drug Administration (FDA) announced on August 14, 2000, that it will regulate hospitals engaged in reprocessing SUDs in the same way that it regulates device manufacturers.

We strongly encourage you to read the "Guidance on Enforcement Priorities for Single-Use Devices Reprocessed by Third Parties and Hospitals," because it describes in detail the requirements of the reuse policy. The document is available at *www.fda.gov/cdrh/comp/guidance/1168.pdf*.

Frequently Asked Questions

Question	Answer
Are all healthcare facilities that reprocess SUDs subject to the requirements?	At this time, FDA is limiting its focus to **hospital** and third-party reprocessors. In the future, FDA will examine whether other establishments that reprocess SUDs should be included.
Does the SUD enforcement guidance apply to all reprocessed SUDs?	It does not apply to<ul><li>permanently implantable pacemakers.</li><li>"open-but-unused" single-use devices.</li><li>hemodialyzers. The reuse of hemodialyzers is addressed in "Guidance for Hemodialyzer Reuse Labeling" of October 6, 1995, at *www.fda.gov/cdrh/ode/dilreuse.pdf*.</li></ul>
Which devices are known to be reprocessed?	Some examples of reprocessed SUDs are surgical saw blades, balloon angioplasty (PTCA) catheters, laparoscopy scissors, and endotracheal tubes. For the complete list of SUDs known to be reprocessed, see Appendix A of the guidance.
What are the regulatory requirements under the Food, Drug, and Cosmetic Act that hospitals must meet if they reprocess SUDs?	The regulatory requirements include<ul><li>establishment registration and device listing (*21 Code of Federal Regulations* (***CFR***) Part 807)</li><li>good manufacturing practice (GMP) under the Quality System regulation (21 ***CFR*** 820)</li><li>device labeling (21 ***CFR*** Part 801)</li><li>submission of adverse events reports under the Medical Device Reporting (MDR) regulation (21 ***CFR*** 803)</li></ul>

Infection Control Compliance Guide: Understanding the JCAHO's Standards

CHAPTER FOUR

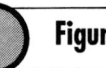

Figure 4.1 — REPROCESSING OF SINGLE-USE MEDICAL DEVICES BY HOSPITALS (CONT.)

Question	Answer
	- medical device tracking (21 *CFR* Part 821) - corrections and removals (21 *CFR* Part 806) - premarket requirements (21 *CFR* Parts 807 and 814)
What is good manufacturing practice under the Quality System regulation?	Hospitals that reprocess SUDs must meet the Quality System (QS) regulation for medical devices (21 *CFR* Part 820). The QS regulation requires a reprocessing hospital to have a quality assurance program or quality system that is appropriate for the specific type of device being reprocessed and that meets the requirements of the QS regulation. FDA monitors compliance with the QS regulation during inspection of the facility. All registered hospitals that reprocess SUDs will be subject to periodic FDA inspection. The requirements under the QS regulation are intended to ensure that continuing quality is incorporated into the devices during reprocessing, rather than by testing and removing defective devices to achieve quality. For more information, see *www.fda.gov/cdrh/dsma/cgmphome.html*.
When must a hospital that reprocesses SUDs meet the regulatory requirements?	For hospital reprocessors, FDA is allowing a one year phase-in period for active enforcement of the **non-premarket** requirements. FDA intends to enforce **premarket submission requirements** by: - February 14, 2001, for **class III** devices - August 14, 2001, for non-exempt **class II** devices - February 14, 2002, for non-exempt **class I** devices
What are class I, II, and III devices?	In general, the *CFR* designates a three-tiered device classification system. Class III devices are generally considered to pose the greatest potential risk to the health of the public and require the most regulation, while class I devices pose the lowest potential risk and require the least regulation. A device's classification is available in 21 *CFR* Parts 862-892 or by searching FDA's database at *www.accessdata.fda.gov/scripts/cdrh/cfdocs/cfpcd/classification.cfm*.

STRATEGIES TO ACHIEVE IC GOALS

Figure 4.1 — REPROCESSING OF SINGLE-USE MEDICAL DEVICES BY HOSPITALS (CONT.)

Question	Answer
How do I know which premarket regulatory requirements apply to my reprocessed device?	The device classification of a reprocessed SUD determines if, when and what type of premarket submission is required. • If your reprocessed SUD is classified as **class I or class II and is exempt**, no premarket submission is required. • If your reprocessed SUD is classified as **class I or class II and is not exempt**, a premarket notification, known as a 510(k), is required. • If your reprocessed SUD is classified as **class III**, generally a premarket approval application, known as a PMA, is required.
How do I register and list reprocessed SUDs?	A hospital that reprocesses SUDs must register with FDA and list every type of reprocessed device. For additional information, see "CDRH Guidance for Industry: Instructions for Completion of Medical Device Registration and Listing Forms FDA-2891, 2891a and 2892" at *www.fda.gov/cdrh/dsma/rlman.html*
What is required for device labeling?	FDA has general labeling requirements regarding the name and place of manufacture and inclusion of adequate directions for use. See "Labeling Regulatory Requirements for Medical Devices" at *www.fda.gov/cdrh/dsma/470.pdf*.
How do I report an adverse event with an SUD?	Hospitals that reprocess SUDs are subject to the manufacturer reporting requirements as well as the user facility reporting requirements (21 *CFR* 803 Subpart E). In addition, they must also adhere to the user facility reporting requirements for all other medical devices that they use. See guidance documents on MDR at *www.fda.gov/cdrh/mdr.html*.
What is "device tracking" and how will a hospital know when to track an SUD?	A hospital that reprocesses SUDs is **not** subject to the Medical Device Tracking regulation (21 *CFR* Part 821) **unless and until** FDA issues a direct order to track a specific device being reprocessed. See "Guidance on Medical Device Tracking" at *www.fda.gov/cdrh/modact/tracking.pdf*
If there are problems with certain reprocessed SUDs and they are removed from inventory, must FDA be notified?	A hospital that reprocesses SUDs must report to FDA, within a specified time, certain types of device corrections and removals. The terms "correction" and "removal" are defined in 21 *CFR* 806.2(3) and 806.2(i).

CHAPTER FOUR

> **Figure 4.1**   **REPROCESSING OF SINGLE-USE MEDICAL DEVICES BY HOSPITALS (CONT.)**
>
> | Question | Answer |
> |---|---|
> | *Need more information?* | In addition to the guidance documents and resources referenced in this brochure, see FDA's Reuse Homepage at *www.fda.gov/cdrh/reuse/index.shtml*. This web site also includes a list of sterility and cleaning standards and related documents for medical devices. To contact FDA's Division of Small Manufacturers Assistance (DSMA), call 301-443-6597 or 1-800-638-2041 or send an e-mail to *dsma@cdrh.fda.gov*. Requests for publications may be submitted by e-mail or by FAX to 301-443-8818. You also are encouraged to visit **Device Advice** at *www.fda.gov/cdrh/devadvice/*. |

- appropriate use of personal protective equipment
    — CDC *Draft—Guideline for Isolation Precautions: Preventing Transmission of Infectious Agents in Healthcare Settings*, 2004 (see below)

c. Implementation of applicable precautions as appropriate are based on the following:
- **The potential for transmission**
- **The mechanism of transmission**
- **The care setting**
- **The emergence and reemergence of pathogens in the community that could affect the hospital**

Most IC programs base their use of precautions on the CDC's recommendations. The CDC's Guidelines for Isolation Precautions in Hospitals (1996) is very detailed in outlining standard-and transmission-based precautions. Put the precautions in place as published or modify for a specific environment.

In June 2004, the CDC published a new draft isolation guideline, titled *Draft—Guideline for Isolation Precautions: Preventing Transmission of Infectious Agents in Healthcare Settings*. When finalized, it will be available at *www.cdc.gov*.

STRATEGIES TO ACHIEVE IC GOALS

d. Screening for exposure/immunity to infectious diseases that LIPs, staff, student/trainees, and volunteers may come in contact within their work is available as warranted.

e. Referral for assessment, potential testing, immunization and/or prophylaxis/treatment, and counseling as appropriate of LIPs, staff, students/trainees, and volunteers who are identified as potentially having an infectious disease or risk of infectious disease that may put the population they serve at risk.

(See Figure 4.2 "Bloodborne Pathogens—Post-Exposure Evaluation & Follow-up Policy," Figure 4.3 "Bloodborne Pathogens—Post-Exposure Evaluation & Follow-up Form," and Figure 4.4 "Bloodborne Pathogens—Post-exposure Evaluation/Healthcare Professional's Written Opinion.")

f. Referral for assessment, potential testing, immunization and/or prophylaxis/treatment, and counseling as appropriate of patients, students/trainees, and volunteers who have been exposed to infectious disease(s) at the hospital and LIPs or staff who are occupationally exposed.

National standards guide the IC aspects of a hospital's occupational health program. In addition, OSHA regulations govern some occupational health activities. Resources that may facilitate compliance with these occupational health standards include the following:

- OSHA Bloodborne Pathogens regulations—1910.1030 (*www.osha.gov/pls/oshaweb/owadisp.show_document?p_table=STANDARDS&p_id=10051*)
- CDC Guidelines for Infection Control in Health Care Personnel, 1998 (*www.cdc.gov/ncidod/hip/guide/infectcont+98.htm*)
- Epidemiology and Prevention of Vaccine-Preventable Diseases (The Pink Book), Advisory Committee on Immunization Practices (*www.cdc.gov/nip/publications/pink/default.htm*)
- "Updated U.S. Public Health Service Guidelines for the Management of Occupational Exposure to HBV, HCV and HIV and Recommendations for Postexposure Prophylaxis," MMWR, 50, no. RR-11 (June 29, 2001).

It is important that the IC components of the occupational health program reflect OSHA regulations

Chapter Four

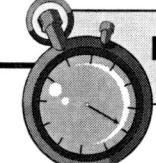

Figure 4.2 Bloodborne Pathogens—Post-Exposure Evaluation & Follow-up Policy

1. First Aid:

At the time of a suspected exposure, basic first aid measures should be taken to thoroughly irrigate and disinfect the affected body part to prevent infection/illness:

   A. Skin exposure, puncture, or laceration – Wash with bactericidal soap and water.

   B. Eyes, mouth or other mucous membranes – Rinse with running water, normal saline, or other suitable sterile eye wash for at least ten (10) minutes.

   Healthcare Workers exposed to HIV, HBV, or HCV being evaluated for exposure or needlestick should be evaluated within hours (rather than days) of their exposure, as HIV Post-exposure prophylaxis (PEP), Hepatitis B vaccine, and HBIG are most effective when administered as soon as possible after exposure.

   C. Rapid screening tests are now available to allow for HIV testing results within hours. This screening test may be followed up with an HIV antibody test as confirmation.

   D. Post-exposure prophylaxis (PEP) is now available, recommended for use after different types of exposures, based on risk of HIV infection.

      1. Risk of type of exposure should be weighed against potential toxicity of PEP.

The healthcare facility should have drugs available for the initial PEP treatment for immediate use.

Employee should be evaluated as soon as possible by a practitioner skilled in use of antiretroviral drugs as well as HIV.

NOTE: Smaller facilities may choose to refer their employees to a hospital/program able to meet these specialized requirements in a timely manner.

Healthcare worker should receive post-exposure counseling, testing and evaluation whether or not PEP is given. Use of condoms/sexual abstinence will be recommended to prevent possible secondary transmission until HIV results are finalized.

Monitoring of PEP toxicity with management should be in place.

Hepatitis B management: see separate policy.

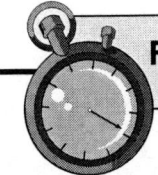

Figure 4.2   BLOODBORNE PATHOGENS—POST-EXPOSURE EVALUATION & FOLLOW-UP POLICY

Hepatitis C Management:

    A. Source patient testing for anti-HCV.

    B. Exposed person:

        2. Baseline testing for anti-HCV and ALT activity.

        3. Follow-up testing (e.g.: 4–6 months) for anti-HCV and ALT activity. Testing for HCV RNA may be substituted for earlier diagnosis.

        4. Confirm all anti-HCV results reported positive by enzyme immunoassay using supplemental anti-HCV testing.

    NOTE: Smaller facilities may choose to refer to acute care facility or skilled practitioner for follow-up.

Source: *CDC, MMWR. "Updated Public Health Service Guidelines for the Management of Occupational Exposures to HBV, HCV and HIV and Recommendations for Postexposure Prophylaxis."* 6/29/2001/Vol. 50/No. RR-11.

and current recommendations of the United States Public Health Service. Find the OSHA regulations and the public health service recommendations on the following Web sites:

- *www.cdc.gov*
- *www.osha.gov*
- *www.niosh.gov*
- *www.cdc.gov/mmwr*

g. Reduction of risks associated with animals brought into the hospital.

Develop a policy on animals brought into your facility. In addition to allowing service animals, some hospitals allow animals in the facility for pet therapy and as adjuncts to the design and furnishings of the hospital environment (e.g., fish tanks and an aviary).

See Figure 4.5 on page 50 for a sample policy on animals in the hospital.

CHAPTER FOUR

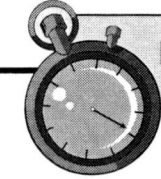

Figure 4.3   PATHOGENS—POST-EXPOSURE EVALUATION & FOLLOW-UP FORM

NOTE: The information on this form is confidential and shall not be released without written permission of the source patient and employee.

Date of Exposure:

Date of Evaluation:

I. Incident Assessment

PART A- *(Part A to be completed by Employee)*

Name of Employee:

Date:

Department:

How did exposure occur? (Include duties leading to exposure.)

Was a sharp involved? (If yes, complete the "sharps injury log".)	❏ Yes	❏ No

Was sharp:	❏ Clean	❏ Contaminated

Severity of Exposure

PART B   *(Part B to be completed by Employee Health Nurse)*

Did significant incident occur?	❏ Yes	❏ No

Signature of Employee Health Nurse	Date:

If exposure is validated, continue on next page

STRATEGIES TO ACHIEVE IC GOALS

Figure 4.3   PATHOGENS—POST-EXPOSURE EVALUATION & FOLLOW-UP FORM (CONT.)

II.	Source
	Patient Assessment - (by Infection Control Practitioner)

Name:	Room #
MR#:	MD:

Current Diagnosis:

Check patient's chart for history of: (Check if positive)

a.	Drug Addiction	☐
b.	Homosexuality	☐
c.	Multiple blood transfusions	☐
d.	HIV Infection	☐
e.	Elevated liver enzymes	☐
f.	Hepatitis B	☐
g.	Hepatitis C	☐

HIV Antibody	Date:	Results:
Hepatitis B Surface Antigen:	Date:	Results:
Anti-HCV:	Date:	Results:

Have a Hepatitis B Surface Antigen, an anti-HCV, and an HIV done on the source *patient if status is unknown or previously negative. Obtain consent.*

III.	Employee Health Office Evaluation and Follow-Up of Employee
	A. Routine Treatment

1. Wound Treated:	Date:	Rx:
By Whom:		

B. Specific Evaluation of Employee

1. History of viral hepatitis:	Type:	Date of diagnosis:
2. Documented evidence of positive Hepatitis B surface antibodies: ☐Yes ☐No		Date:
3. Hepatitis B Vaccine?	Year:	# of doses:

** If all of these questions are <u>NO</u> - proceed...

Infection Control Compliance Guide: Understanding the JCAHO's Standards

CHAPTER FOUR

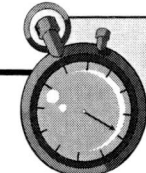

Figure 4.3 — PATHOGENS—POST-EXPOSURE EVALUATION & FOLLOW-UP FORM (CONT.)

	4. Test for Hepatitis B surface antibody:		Date:	Results:
	5. Refer to HBV post-exposure algorithm.			
C.	HIV Status - Employee			
	1. HIV status known:		Date of evaluation:	
	2. Discuss HIV testing and follow-up protocol			
	3. Have consent signed and perform test as soon as feasible after exposure			
	Date:		By whom:	
	Refer to Potential HIV Exposure protocol for follow-up testing.			
	If employee refuses test, notify the Laboratory to freeze baseline blood for 90 days - test at any time if employee gives consent.			
D.	HCV Evaluation – Employee			
	1. Get an anti-HCV and ALT on the employee.			
	Employee HCV: Date:		Results:	
	ALT Date:		Results:	
	2. If negative, repeat anti-HCV and ALT in 6 months.			
	3. Confirm by supplemental anti-HCV testing of all anti-HCV results reported as positive by enzyme immunoassay.			
E.	Notify employee to report any acute viral illnesses during the next three (3) months.			
	❑ Yes	❑ No	Date:	
F.	If employee's initial HIV test is negative, and the source patient's is positive, retest as follows:			
		Date Of Consent	**Test Results**	
	6 weeks:			
	3 months			
	6 months:			
G.	Follow-up appointment			
	Date		Time	
H.	Health Care Professional's written opinion of evaluation:			
		1. _____(name) is to complete Healthcare Professional's written opinion.		
		2. Obtain employee's signature and file the completed forms in employee's Medical Record.		

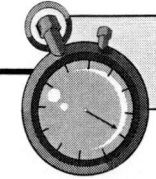

Figure 4.4 — Bloodborne Pathogens Post-Exposure Evaluation / Healthcare Professional's Written Option

NOTE: Prior to the evaluation, the healthcare professional will be provided—
1. A copy of the OSHA standard on bloodborne pathogens
2. A description of the exposed employee's duties as they relate to the exposure incident.
3. Documentation of the route of exposure and circumstances under which exposure occurred.
4. Results of the source individual's blood testing.
5. Relevant medical records including vaccination status.

This requirement will be met by providing the healthcare professional with the completed form, "Post-Exposure Evaluation and Follow-Up."

WRITTEN OPINION

I have assessed _____ on _____
                     employee   date
for an exposure incident which occurred on _____.
                                            date

❑ I have a copy of the 1999 OSHA standard, the "Post-Exposure Evaluation and Follow-Up" form from the employer and a copy of the 2001 USPHS Recommendations for Hepatitis B prophylaxis Following Percutaneous or Permucosal Exposure.

I.	**HEPATITIS B IMMUNIZATION (Check one)**	
	❑ Hepatitis prophylaxis is indicated.	❑ Hepatitis B prophylaxis is not indicated.
II.	**HEPATITIS C TESTING/EVALUATION FOLLOW-UP.** ❑ Indicated ❑ Not Indicated	
III.	**POST EXPOSURE EVALUATION AND FOLLOW-UP (Check all that apply)**	
	The employee has been informed of the results of my evaluation.	❑
	The employee has been informed of any medical conditions resulting from exposure to blood or other potentially infectious materials which require further evaluation or treatment.	❑

Signature of Healthcare Professional	Date
Signature of Exposed Employee	Date
Witness of Employee's Signature	

This form must be received by the employer and a copy provided to the employee within 15 days of the evaluation.

CHAPTER FOUR

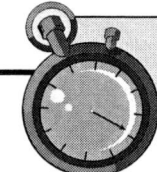

Figure 4.5   ANIMALS IN THE HOSPITAL POLICY

PURPOSE:

To ensure that animals used for pet therapy and service animals pose no danger to the patients.

POLICY:

X. General infection control measures for animal encounters

    E. Contact with animal saliva, dander, urine, and feces will be minimized.

    F. Hand hygiene will be practiced after any animal contact.

XI. Animal-assisted activities and resident animal programs:

    A. Selection of nonhuman primates and reptiles in animal-assisted activities, animal-assisted therapy, or resident animal programs will be avoided.

    B. Animals that are fully vaccinated for zoonotic diseases and that are healthy, clean, well-groomed, and negative for enteric parasites or otherwise have completed recent anthelmintic treatment under the regular care of a veterinarian will be used in the program.

    C. Animals that are trained with the assistance or under the direction of persons who are experienced in this field will be used in the program.

    D. Animals will be controlled by persons trained in providing activities or therapies safely, and who know the animal's health status and behavior traits.

    E. Prompt action will be taken when an incident of biting or scratching by an animal occurs during an animal-assisted activity or therapy.

        1. The animal will be removed permanently from these programs.

        2. The incident will be reported promptly to appropriate authorities (e.g., infection-control staff, animal program coordinator, or local animal control personnel).

        3. Bites, scratches or other breaks in the skin will be promptly treated and cleaned.

    F. An infection control risk assessment will be completed before conducting an animal-assisted activity or therapy to determine whether the session should be held in a public area of the facility or in individual patient rooms.

    G. Precautions to mitigate allergic responses to animals will be taken.

        1. Shedding of animal dander will be minimized by bathing animals less than 24 hours before a visit.

        2. Either animals will be groomed to remove loose hair before a visit or a therapy animal cape will be used.

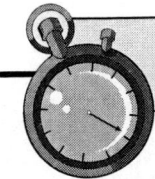

Figure 4.5 — Animals in the Hospital Policy (cont.)

H. Routine cleaning protocols for housekeeping surfaces will be used after therapy sessions.

I. Resident animals, including fish in tanks, will be restricted from access to patient-care areas, food preparation areas, dining areas, laundry areas, central sterile supply areas, sterile and clean supply storage areas, medication preparation areas, operating rooms, isolation areas, and PE areas.

J. Facility policy will be established for regular cleaning of fish tanks, rodent cages, and bird cages, and any other animal dwellings. This cleaning task will be assigned to a non-patient-care staff member; splashing tank water or contaminating environmental surfaces with animal bedding will be avoided.

XII. Protective measures for immunocompromised patients

A. Patients will be advised to avoid contact with animal feces, saliva, urine, or solid litter box material.

B. Scratches, bites, or other wounds that break the skin will be promptly cleaned and treated.

C. Patients will be advised to avoid direct or indirect contact with reptiles.

D. Case-by-case assessment will be conducted to determine whether animal-assisted activities or animal-assisted therapy programs are appropriate for immunocompromised patients.

XIII. Service animals

A. Providing facility access to nonhuman primates and reptiles as service animals will be avoided.

B. Service animals will be allowed access to the facility in accordance with the Americans with Disabilities Act of 1990, unless the presence of the animal creates a direct threat to other persons or a fundamental alteration in the nature of services. (U.S. Department of Justice: 28 CFR § 36.302)

C. When a decision must be made regarding a service animal's access to any particular area of the healthcare facility, the service animal, patient, and healthcare situation will be evaluated on a case-by-case basis to determine whether significant risk of harm exists and whether reasonable modifications in policies and procedures will mitigate this risk. (U.S. Department of Justice: 28 CFR § 36.302)

D. If a patient must be separated from his or her service animal while in the healthcare facility, 1) staff will ascertain from the person what arrangements have been made for supervision or care of the animal during this period of separation and 2) appropriate arrangements will be made to address the patient's needs in the absence of the service animal.

Source: HCPro Infection Control Manual for Hospitals

CHAPTER FIVE

Effectiveness of IC interventions

> **Review of the standard:**
>
> **IC.5.10** The infection control (IC) program evaluates the effectiveness of the infection control interventions and, as necessary, redesigns the infection control interventions.

This chapter provides information on evaluating the effectiveness of IC interventions and presents a format for testing those strategies.

> **How to survey the standard:**
> - Interview IC staff
>
> **Documents that may be requested or reviewed:**
> - Written IC plan/evaluation of effectiveness

Elements of performance for IC.5.10

> 1. The hospital formally evaluates and revises the goals and program (or portions of the program) at least annually and whenever risks are significantly changed.

Complete at least annually a formal evaluation of your hospital's IC risks, goals, and interventions. Conduct interim evaluations when changes emerge in the risks relating to infections.

CHAPTER FIVE

In many hospitals, IC staff conduct the initial evaluation of the IC program's effectiveness with input from departmental leaders and others as needed. After doing so, IC staff should present their evaluation to both leadership and the IC committee for input. Consider assigning the IC committee or a task force of persons knowledgeable about a specific goal to redesign the strategy and to present the revision back to the IC committee.

> **2. The evaluation addresses**

- **changes in the scope of the IC program (e.g., resulting from the introduction of new services or new sites of care)**
- **changes in the results of the IC program risk analysis**

Address in the evaluation any new services (e.g., transplant); new sites of care (e.g., new outpatient surgery center and satellite hospitals); major construction or renovation projects; and other changes that could modify risk to the patient population.

> **3. The evaluation addresses emerging and reemerging problems in the healthcare community that potentially affect the hospital (e.g., highly infectious agents).**

Include in the evaluation initial cases of emerging infectious diseases (e.g., avian influenza), threats of biologic-weapons use in the community, new or changing patterns of resistant organisms, and other community issues. These situations could occur at any time and could trigger an interim evaluation of the IC plan.

> **4. The evaluation addresses the assessment of the success or failure of interventions for preventing and controlling infection.**

To determine the success of the strategies, include an assessment of your evaluation methods in your IC plan. Monitor the effectiveness of your interventions on an ongoing basis and determine at least annually whether your strategies need to be revised. See Figure 5.1 on page 55 to assess the strategies and interventions in place at your facility.

Figure 5.1 — **TESTING OF STRATEGIES**

TESTING OF STRATEGIES

Use this form to assess the strategies and interventions in place in your facility.

Strategy	Goal Addressed	Questions to Ask	Answer
(EXAMPLE) Placement of alcohol handrub in every patient room	Appropriate hand hygiene in direct patient care	Is it reasonable?	☐ Yes ☐ No
		Does it accurately address the risk that has been identified?	☐ Yes ☐ No
		Is it feasible?	☐ Yes ☐ No
		Can it be accomplished within the specific hospital environment?	☐ Yes ☐ No
		Is it cost-effective?	☐ Yes ☐ No
		If it is not cost-effective, do the benefits that may be derived outweigh the costs?	☐ Yes ☐ No
		Is it reasonable?	☐ Yes ☐ No
		Does it accurately address the risk that has been identified?	☐ Yes ☐ No
		Is it feasible?	☐ Yes ☐ No
		Can it be accomplished within the specific hospital environment?	☐ Yes ☐ No
		Is it cost-effective?	☐ Yes ☐ No
		If it is not cost-effective, do the benefits that may be derived outweigh the costs?	☐ Yes ☐ No
		Is it reasonable?	☐ Yes ☐ No
		Does it accurately address the risk that has been identified?	☐ Yes ☐ No
		Is it feasible?	☐ Yes ☐ No
		Can it be accomplished within the specific hospital environment?	☐ Yes ☐ No
		Is it cost-effective?	☐ Yes ☐ No
		If it is not cost-effective, do the benefits that may be derived outweigh the costs?	☐ Yes ☐ No
		Is it reasonable?	☐ Yes ☐ No
		Does it accurately address the risk that has been identified?	☐ Yes ☐ No
		Is it feasible?	☐ Yes ☐ No
		Can it be accomplished within the specific hospital environment?	☐ Yes ☐ No
		Is it cost-effective?	☐ Yes ☐ No
		If it is not cost-effective, do the benefits that may be derived outweigh the costs?	☐ Yes ☐ No

Chapter Five

> **5. The evaluation addresses responses to concerns raised by leadership and others within the hospital.**

Immediately address any significant concerns—from leadership or from others in the hospital—that arise during the evaluation. Consider integrating these concerns into the overall evaluation of the IC program, especially if they were legitimate concerns that required action.

> **6. The evaluation addresses the evolution of relevant infection prevention and control guidelines that are based on evidence or, in the absence of evidence, expert consensus.**

You and your staff should be aware of changes to pertinent IC guidelines, recommendations, and standards of practice. Assess in a timely manner new recommendations—especially Centers for Disease Control and Prevention (CDC) Category 1 recommendations—to determine whether the program's strategies need to be revised to align with new evidence-based guidelines.

The CDC provides occasional, time-sensitive e-mails about important healthcare events (e.g., outbreaks, product recalls) and publications (e.g., new healthcare guidelines) to persons interested in the prevention of healthcare-acquired infections and antimicrobial resistance. There is no charge for the service. Subscribe to its rapid notification system at *http://www2a.cdc.gov/ncidod/hip/rns/hip_rns_subscribe.html*.

CHAPTER SIX

Influx of infectious patients

> ### Review of the standard:
> **IC.6.10** As part of emergency management activities, the organization prepares to respond to an influx, or the risk of an influx, of infectious patients.

This chapter prepares you to comply with the new standard for planning your facility's response to an influx, or risk of influx, of infectious patients; determining methods of obtaining current information; disseminating information; and identifying community resources.

> **How to survey the standard:**
> - Interview IC staff
> - Interview staff
> - Interview safety officer
>
> **Documents that may be requested or reviewed:**
> - Emergency management plan
> - Emergency/disaster drills
> - IC policies and procedures

CHAPTER SIX

Elements of performance for IC.6.10

> 1. The organization plans its response to an influx, or risk of an influx, of infectious patients.
>
> 2. The organization has a plan for managing an influx of potentially infectious patients/residents/clients over an extended period of time.

Multiple factors and community events could lead to an influx of infectious patients into your hospital. Examples include the following:
- A natural community outbreak of an infectious disease that causes serious morbidity (e.g., influenza requiring hospitalization)
- Multiple cases of infectious disease following a bioterrorism event (e.g., widespread anthrax or smallpox exposure)
- Referrals from other healthcare facilities experiencing a widespread outbreak and needing isolation rooms for patients

Your facility should create specific written plans regarding your response to an influx, or risk of influx, of infectious patients. Make the plan a part of your current emergency management plan (see figure 6.1 for a sample policy). It should describe how to
- provide safe transport of patients to your hospital
- triage new patients
- provide safe transport of patients within your hospital
- set up common space for grouping infectious patients, if needed (temporarily or for an extended period of time)
- establish methods to set up controlled environments (e.g., negative pressure), if required by the specific disease
- create communication networks
 — within the facility
 — with appropriate community resources and emergency management systems
 — with the public and the news media

> 3. The organization

- **determines how it will keep abreast of current information about the emergence of epidemics or new infections that may result in the organization activating its response**

INFLUX OF INFECTIOUS PATIENTS

The following is a list of resources that can help you keep current on the emergence of epidemics/new infections state- and nation-wide:
- The CDC's Morbidity and Mortality Weekly Report (www.cdc.gov/mmwr/)
- Infectious disease reports from state epidemiology offices
- Communication with local public health departments
- The CDC's rapid notification system (http://www2a.cdc.gov/ncidod/hip/rns/hip_rns_subscribe.html)
- The Association for Professionals in Infection Control and Epidemiology/state organization networks

Determine other resources available within your county as well.

- **determines how it will disseminate critical information to staff and other key practitioners**

Plan ahead for disseminating information to staff when there is an increase in the numbers of patients with infectious diseases. Consider the following methods:
- E-mail messages to staff/managers with on-the-job access to e-mail
- Post bulletins near time clocks, in break rooms, and in other areas staff frequent
- Distribute daily newsletters to departments/units

- **identifies resources in the community (through local, state, and/or federal public health systems) for obtaining additional information**

Maintain a list of pertinent community/state/national resources, including the following:
- Local public health departments
- State epidemiology
- Civil defense
- Local emergency management services
- Federal Bureau of Investigation

Infection Control Compliance Guide: Understanding the JCAHO's Standards

Chapter Six

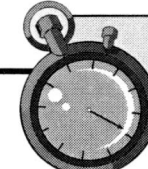

Figure 6.1 — Influx of People with Infectious Diseases Policy

In addition to implementation of the general Emergency Management policies, the following issues will be addressed for infectious diseases.

COMMUNITY RESOURCES

Determine if this is a community-wide event and if other facilities, shelters, hotels, etc. are also accepting the infectious patients. If so, coordinate decision-making with community disaster agencies and local/state public health departments.

TYPE OF INFECTIOUS DISEASE/MODE OF TRANSMISSION

Determine what types of infectious disease the patients have and its mode of transmission. If the mode of transmission is any mode that requires precautions beyond standard precautions, make a decision regarding the following:

1. Are rooms needed with negative pressure for isolation?

    If yes, does the facility have adequate negative pressure rooms or can rooms be retrofitted for negative pressure?

    Can several patients fit into the available negative pressure rooms and thus accommodate the influx?

    Can a wing of the building that does not share an air system with the rest of the building be used for the infectious patients?

    Does the entire building need to be emptied of patients without the infectious disease so the building can be used for only patients with the infectious disease?

    Does an outdoor temporary shelter need to be implemented to house the infectious patients?

2. If negative pressure is not needed but contact or droplet precautions are,

    Does the facility have adequate rooms/spaces to cohort the patients with the infectious disease?

    Does the building or a section of the building need to be emptied of the less ill patients to accommodate those with the infectious disease?

    Is the influx so large that a temporary shelter needs to be implemented for the infectious patients?

SUPPLIES

Are adequate supplies available for personal protective equipment and hand hygiene? If not, initiate ordering the necessary supplies.

STAFFING FOR THE INFECTIOUS PATIENTS

If this is a disease for which some healthcare workers have immunity, consider if there is a need to assign those staff with immunity to care for the infectious patients.

MEDICATIONS FOR TREATMENT AND PROPHYLAXIS

If there is an indication for specific drug treatment of the infectious patients and/or prophylaxis for exposed persons, initiate the process for obtaining those medications in adequate quantity.

Note: Implementation of this guideline will be in conjunction with other measures identified in the Emergency Management Plan including triage, staffing, communication, visitors, news media, food/water, etc.

CHAPTER SEVEN

Effective management of the IC program

Review of the standard:
IC.7.10 The infection control (IC) program is managed effectively.

This chapter reviews the standard that requires effective management of your program. It addresses the qualifications and competency of individuals responsible for managing the IC program. It also provides an IC competency assessment for use either as a self-assessment or as your facility's formal competency assessment for the infection control professional (ICP).

How to survey the standard:
- Interview IC staff
- Interview leadership

Documents that may be requested or reviewed:
- Written IC plan
- Competency records

Elements of performance for IC.7.10

> 1. The hospital assigns responsibility for managing IC program activities to one or more individuals whose number, competency, and skill mix are determined by the goals and objectives of the IC activities.

Your hospital's written IC plan should clearly identify the goals, objectives, and priorities of the IC program. The surveyors will likely review the IC plan to determine whether adequate numbers of IC staff are available to meet the program's goals and objectives.

In addition, the competency and skill mix of the IC staff should reflect the complexity of the facility. For example, if a hospital has a transplant program, one or more members of the IC staff should have knowledge/competency of infection prevention in the immunocompromised host (see Figure 7.1 on page 63 for an IC competency assessment checklist).

Figure 7.1 — Infection Control Competency Assessment

To perform a self-assessment of competence and qualifications for the infection control position, complete the following. Score each area with

1 = competent
2 = needs improvement
3 = not competent

Management

Has knowledge of				Actions to address (scores of 2 or 3)
basic principles of management	1	2	3	
the steps in the problem-solving process	1	2	3	
concepts of change theory	1	2	3	

Education

Has knowledge of				Actions to address (scores of 2 or 3)
principles of adult education	1	2	3	
conducting a needs/knowledge assessment of the learners	1	2	3	
educational techniques and methods for adults	1	2	3	
learner evaluation techniques	1	2	3	
teaching strategies	1	2	3	

Surveillance

Has knowledge of				Actions to address (scores of 2 or 3)
principles of epidemiology	1	2	3	
surveillance methods	1	2	3	
criteria for healthcare-associated infections	1	2	3	
Basic statistical calculations	1	2	3	

Figure 7.1 — INFECTION CONTROL COMPETENCY ASSESSMENT (CONT.)

Data display				
Reporting mechanisms	1	2	3	

Outbreak detection and management

Has knowledge of				Actions to address (scores of 2 or 3)
steps in an outbreak investigation	1	2	3	
detection of trends, clusters, outbreaks	1	2	3	
state reporting requirements	1	2	3	
methods to obtain assistance	1	2	3	

Policies and procedures

Has knowledge of				Actions to address (scores of 2 or 3)
organization's policy/procedure format	1	2	3	
Has ability to				
develop an appropriately constructed policy/procedure based on appropriate evidence-based/standards of practice	1	2	3	

Consultation for infection control

Has knowledge of				Actions to address (scores of 2 or 3)
effective methods of communication	1	2	3	

Has access to				Actions to address (scores of 2 or 3)
appropriate knowledge resources (textbooks, journals, web)	1	2	3	

Collaboration with departments, functions, and services

Has knowledge of				Actions to address (scores of 2 or 3)
department managers within the organization	1	2	3	

Figure 7.1 — INFECTION CONTROL COMPETENCY ASSESSMENT (CONT.)

organizational leadership	1	2	3
service chiefs	1	2	3
committees/teams	1	2	3

Infection control aspects of occupational health

Has knowledge of				Actions to address (scores of 2 or 3)
occupational health/IC policies and procedures	1	2	3	
occupational health/IC processes	1	2	3	
regulatory requirements	1	2	3	

Qualifications	Yes	No
Attendance at a basic training program for infection control and epidemiology	1	2
Structural mentoring by an experienced ICP		
Certification in IC	1	2
If in the field less than two years, preparing for certification	1	2
Established a network of other infection control professionals	1	2
Participates in ongoing inservices	1	2
Participates in meetings/conferences specific to infection control/epidemiology	1	2

Chapter Seven

> **2. Qualifications of the individual(s) responsible for managing the IC program are determined by the risks entailed in the services provided, the hospital's patient population(s), and the complexity of the activities that will be carried out.**

Note: **Qualifications may be met through ongoing education, training, experience, and/or certification (e.g., Certification Board for Infection Control [CBIC] in the prevention and control of infections).**

Surveyors routinely focus on the qualifications of IC staff. A specific degree or educational background is not required, but you must document your IC staff's basic qualifications (e.g., in nursing, as a medical technologist, etc.) as well as evidence of ongoing educational opportunities. Options for these opportunities include

- attending a basic training program for IC and epidemiology
- working with an experienced ICP as a mentor (which is especially important if the new ICP is in a rural area with limited access to training)
- gaining knowledge through experience in the field of IC/epidemiology
- attending intermediate or advanced training programs
- participating in ongoing inservice education
- maintaining certification in IC

Qualifications/training should include information pertinent to the patient population, acuity of illness, patient-care technology used, and the risks relating to healthcare-associated infections, as well as general principles of IC and epidemiology. The JCHAO does not specifically mandate certification in IC, but having it is considered the national "gold standard" for experienced ICPs. Many surveyors will question whether your staff are obtaining or pursuing certification.

Document qualifications in personnel files and make them available to surveyors for review.

> **3. This individual(s) coordinates all infection prevention and control within the hospital.**

IC staff should be able to demonstrate involvement in IC activities throughout the organization. They serve as consultants to all services and departments and assist them in decision-making relating to IC issues. They demonstrate their involvement through collaboration with departments on policies and procedures, feedback of IC data to departments (when warranted), and assistance in problem solving.

EFFECTIVE MANAGEMENT OF THE IC PROGRAM

> **4. This individual(s) facilitates ongoing monitoring of the effectiveness of prevention and/or control activities and interventions.**

Minimally involve your IC staff in oversight roles so they can monitor effectiveness of IC activities/interventions throughout the organization. Some IC staff may choose to take a more active role in monitoring effectiveness of IC interventions. Regardless of how it does so, your IC program should reflect that you have accomplished IC interventions. Incorporate this information into the written IC plan.

CHAPTER EIGHT

Collaboration in implementing the IC program

Review of the standard:

IC.8.10 Representatives from relevant components/functions within the hospital collaborate to implement the infection control (IC) program.

This chapter addresses the need for hospital leaders to work together in establishing and evaluating their IC programs.

How to survey the standard:
- Interview IC staff
- Interview leadership
- Interview department managers

Documents that may be requested or reviewed:
- Written IC plan
- Departmental IC policies and procedures
- IC committee minutes

CHAPTER EIGHT

Elements of Performance for IC.8.10

> 1. Hospital leaders including medical staff, LIPs, and other direct and indirect patient care staff (including, when applicable, pharmacy, laboratory, administration, central supply/sterilization services, housekeeping, building maintenance/engineering, and food services) collaborate on an ongoing basis with the qualified individual(s) managing the IC program.

Since the 1970s, there has been a saying that "Infection control is everyone's responsibility." This JCAHO standard reiterates that principle.

IC cannot be effective if it is the responsibility of only one department. Therefore, involve hospital leaders and direct/indirect patient care staff in putting the IC program in place. Involve leaders in development, implementation, and evaluation of the IC program. Direct patient-care staff will also determine the success or failure of the program. As the group that provides "hands-on" care, they have the potential to directly increase or decrease the risk of infection.

> 2. These representatives participate in the following:

- **Development of strategies for each component's/function's role in the IC program**

  Each component or function within the hospital plays a role in infection prevention and control. Therefore, involve representatives from each service and department in policy and procedure development, review, and revision. Once you determine priorities and goals, involve leaders in developing strategies to accomplish the goals.

- **Assessment of the adequacy of the human, information, physical, and financial resources allocated to support infection prevention and control activities**

  Conduct an ongoing assessment of the adequacy of infection prevention and control resources. The best sources of information for this assessment are IC department's staff.

  IC staff are responsible for making leaders aware of resources needed but not yet available. Leaders then are responsible for assessing these needs and acting based on that assessment. See Chapter nine for more information on resources.

Collaboration in Implementing the IC Program

- **Assessment of the overall failure or success of key processes for preventing and controlling infection**

Hospital leadership should collaborate with the IC program to assess whether the program's goals are being met and the key processes/strategies used to meet them are succeeding.

- **The review and revision of the IC program as warranted to improve outcomes**

Involve leaders in reviewing the program and, if needed, in revising the program's strategies to help you accomplish your goals. Leaders may demonstrate collaboration in the following ways:

- Document attendance at meetings during which they evaluate and revise the IC plan
- Hold meetings with IC staff to review the IC plan
- Provide written feedback to the IC committee after reviewing the plan and its accomplishments
- Sign off on the written IC plan

CHAPTER NINE

Adequate resources for the IC program

> ### Review of the standard:
> **IC.9.10** Hospital leaders allocate adequate resources for the infection control (IC) program.

This chapter discusses the need for hospital leaders to allocate adequate resources for the IC program. It also provides a checklist you can use to evaluate whether your IC program has adequate resources available.

> **How to survey the standard:**
> - Interview leaders
> - Interview IC staff
> - Interview laboratory manager/staff
> - Observation of available resources
>
> **Documents that may be requested or reviewed:**
> - Minutes of the patient safety program
> - IC plan and signatures

An effective IC program is a critical component of patient safety and quality care. Although it is generally not a revenue producing program, the payoff for its effectiveness can be great and may include the following:

Chapter Nine

- Improved patient outcomes
- Decreased patient length of stay and corresponding costs
- Compliance with national recommendations and standards of practice, resulting in improved quality of care and defense against litigation
- Compliance with regulations and accreditation standards
- Enhanced teamwork and collaboration between departments

Elements of Performance for IC.9.10

> **1. Leaders review on an ongoing basis (but no less frequently than annually) the effectiveness of the hospital's infection prevention and control activities and report their findings to the integrated patient safety program.**

At least once a year, leaders should review the IC program. They should then present the findings to the patient safety program.

Many hospitals have liaison positions from the IC committee to the patient safety committees and vice versa. This collaboration enhances the relationship, communication, and reporting between the two committees.

> **2. Adequate systems to access information are provided to support infection prevention and control activities.**
> **3. When applicable, adequate laboratory support is provided to support infection prevention and control activities.**

For an effective IC program, it is critical that you obtain accurate and timely information. Computerization of patient information, including lab data, with easy access for the ICP, can help in this effort and make the IC department more efficient. In fact, acquiring specific data in a timely manner is the core of infection surveillance. Infection prevention and control software can improve an IC department's efficiency in recording, displaying, and reporting infection data as well as performing statistical tests on the data. Software can help you use data by

- allowing you to develop upper and lower thresholds for your site-specific infection data and informing you when data is "out of control" or outside the expected range
- performing tests of significance on data in evaluating an outbreak
- providing data in a visual format for the IC committee's review

Another aspect of having "adequate systems" is providing appropriate man-hours for effective IC. Although there does not yet seem to be a strong national standard for requiring IC full-time equivalents (FTE), the following publications provide guidelines:

- C. O'Boyle, M. Jackson, and S.J. Henly, "Staffing Requirements for Infection Control Programs in U.S. Health Care Facilities: Delphi project." Am J Infect. Control 30, no. 6 (2000): 321–333.

  The Delphi panel recommended a ratio of 0.8 to 1.0 ICP for every 100 occupied beds as adequate staffing.

- Health Canada, Nosocomial and Occupational Infections Section. Development of a resource model for infection prevention and control programs in acute, long term, and home care settings: Conference proceedings of the Infection Prevention and Control Alliance. Am J Infect Control 32 (2003): 2–6.

  The models developed by this group project that an infection prevention and control program needs three FTE IC professionals per 500 beds in acute-care hospitals and one FTE ICP per 150–200 beds in long-term care facilities.

> **4. Adequate equipment and supplies are provided to support infection prevention and control activities.**

Like all other hospital functions/departments, the IC program must have adequate equipment and supplies. Such supplies may include computers, hardware, software, Internet access, and office equipment and supplies.

See Figure 9.1 on page 76 for a checklist of IC resources.

Figure 9.1 — INFECTION CONTROL RESOURCES

Resource	Available Yes	Available No	If no, action needed	Target date
Adequate FTE's for the IC department				
Adequate physical space within the IC department				
Convenient access to patient-specific data (including lab data)				
Knowledge-based information				
• Textbooks				
• Journals				
• Internet access				
• E-learning				
• Training/programs/conferences				
• APIC/state organization meetings				
Collaboration with departments, services, and pertinent committees				
Adequate budget				
Equipment:				
• Computer				
• Printer				
• Facsimile machine				
• Telephone with message services				
• Beeper (if necessary)				
• Basic office supplies				
Software				
• IC/epidemiology software				
• Word processor				
• Database				
• Spreadsheet				
• Presentations				
• Accounting				
• Organizational/flow chart				

Introduction to chapters 10 and 11

The JCAHO National Patient Safety Goals

To promote improvements in patient safety, the Joint Commission on Accreditation of Healthcare Organizations (JCAHO) has developed National Patient Safety Goals. The goals reflect problematic areas in healthcare and describe evidence- and expert-based ways to handle them.

The JCAHO evaluates accredited organizations for continuous compliance with the National Patient Safety Goals and with the JCAHO standards. These requirements tend to be more prescriptive than JCAHO standards requirements, but organizations may design alternative approaches to meeting the goals and to request JCAHO consideration and approval of such alternatives.

The National Patient Safety Goals are developed based on recommendations made in the JCAHO's safety newsletter, *Sentinel Event Alert*. The Sentinel Event Advisory Group works with JCAHO staff to determine priorities for potential safety improvements and to develop goals and specific requirements. Then potential new goals and requirements are sent to the field for review and comment.

The advisory group annually recommends selected existing and new goals and requirements to the JCAHO's Board of Commissioners for final review and approval. The advisory group also assists the JCAHO in evaluating potential alternatives to goal requirements that individual organizations suggest. For example, the JCAHO could approve an alternative method of accomplishing one of the category I CDC hand-hygiene guidelines if it is equally effective.

As for 2004, the JCAHO came out with a goal relating to infection prevention and control for 2005: Goal #7. This goal, which is divided into two parts, reads, "Reduce the risk of healthcare-acquired infections." The first part, Goal #7a, concerns complying with the Centers for Disease Control and Prevention hand-hygiene guidelines. The second part, Goal #7b, deals with managing certain healthcare-acquired infections as sentinel events.

Chapters ten and eleven of this book provide information on Goal #7.

CHAPTER TEN

Hand-hygiene safety goal

This chapter reviews the JCAHO National Patient Safety Goal #7a, which requires compliance with current Centers for Disease Control and Prevention (CDC) hand-hygiene guidelines.

How to survey the goal:
- Interview IC staff
- Interview department managers
- Interview staff
- Observation of practices
- Observation of equipment, handwashing facilities, and hand-hygiene products

Documents that may be requested or reviewed:
- IC policies and procedures
- Compliance documentation

Safety Goal #7: Reduce the risk of healthcare-acquired infections.
Goal #7a: Comply with current CDC hand-hygiene guidelines.

The CDC's hand-hygiene guidelines were published the Guidelines for Hand Hygiene in Health-Care Settings (www.cdc.gov/handhygiene), which appeared in the October 25, 2002 *Morbidity and Mortality Weekly Report*. This document provides specific recommendations to promote improved hand-hygiene practice and to reduce transmission of pathogenic microorganisms to patients and personnel in healthcare settings.

Chapter Ten

The JCAHO incorporated those hand-hygiene guidelines into the National Patient Safety Goals. And although the JCAHO does not require implementation of all the hand-hygiene recommendations, it does require implementation of all Category 1 recommendations, including those in Category 1A, 1B, and 1C (see Figure 10.1 for an explanation of categories). Also, consider implementing Category 11 recommendations, although they are not required for accreditation.

The following list identifies the material contained in Figures 10.1–10.5:
- Figure 10.1 on this page describes the CDC system for categorizing its recommendations
- Figure 10.2 on page 81 lists all of the CDC hand-hygiene recommendations and provides a quick reference that IC programs can use to assess compliance with the Category 1 recommendations
- Figure 10.3 on page 85 provides a sample tool for monitoring hand-hygiene compliance
- Figure 10.4 on page 86 provides a hand-hygiene guidelines fact sheet from the CDC
- Figure 10.5 on page 88 provides a sample hand-hygiene policy

Figure 10.1   CATEGORIES OF CDC RECOMMENDATIONS

Each CDC/HICPAC recommendation is categorized on the basis of existing scientific data, theoretical rationale, applicability, and economic impact. The CDC/HICPAC system for categorizing recommendations is as follows:

Category 1A: Strongly recommended for implementation and strongly supported by well-designed experimental, clinical, or epidemiological studies.

Category 1B: Strongly recommended for implementation and supported by certain experimental, clinical, or epidemiological studies and a strong theoretical rationale.

Category 1C: Required for implementation, as mandated by federal or state regulation or standard.

Category 2: Suggested for implementation and supported by suggestive clinical or epidemiologic studies or a theoretical rationale.

No recommendation. Unresolved issue. Practices for which insufficient evidence or no consensus regarding efficacy exist.

Figure 10.2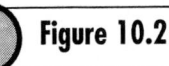

CDC HAND-HYGIENE RECOMMENDATIONS

Note: The references may be accessed at *www.cdc.gov/handhygiene/*

1. Indications for handwashing and hand antisepsis

- When hands are visibly dirty or contaminated with proteinaceous material or are visibly soiled with blood or other body fluids, wash hands with either a non-antimicrobial soap and water or an antimicrobial soap and water (IA) (*66*).

- If hands are not visibly soiled, use an alcohol-based hand rub for routinely decontaminating hands in all other clinical situations described in items 1C—J (IA) (*74,93,166,169,283,294,312,398*). Alternatively, wash hands with an antimicrobial soap and water in all clinical situations described in items 1C—J (IB) (*69-71,74*).

- Decontaminate hands before having direct contact with patients (IB) (*68,400*).

- Decontaminate hands before donning sterile gloves when inserting a central intravascular catheter (IB) (*401,402*).

- Decontaminate hands before inserting indwelling urinary catheters, peripheral vascular catheters, or other invasive devices that do not require a surgical procedure (IB) (*25,403*).

- Decontaminate hands after contact with a patient's intact skin (e.g., when taking a pulse or blood pressure, and lifting a patient) (IB) (*25,45,48,68*).

- Decontaminate hands after contact with body fluids or excretions, mucous membranes, nonintact skin, and wound dressings if hands are not visibly soiled (IA) (*400*).

- Decontaminate hands if moving from a contaminated-body site to a clean-body site during patient care (II) (*25,53*).

- Decontaminate hands after contact with inanimate objects (including medical equipment) in the immediate vicinity of the patient (II) (*46,53,54*).

- Decontaminate hands after removing gloves (IB) (*50,58,321*).

- Before eating and after using a restroom, wash hands with a non-antimicrobial soap and water or with an antimicrobial soap and water (IB) (*404-409*).

- Antimicrobial-impregnated wipes (i.e., towelettes) may be considered as an alternative to washing hands with non-antimicrobial soap and water. Because they are not as effective as alcohol-based hand rubs or washing hands with an antimicrobial soap and water for reducing bacterial counts on the hands of HCWs, they are not a substitute for using an alcohol-based hand rub or antimicrobial soap (IB) (*160,161*).

- Wash hands with non-antimicrobial soap and water or with antimicrobial soap and water if exposure to *Bacillus anthracis* is suspected or proven. The physical action of washing and rinsing hands under such circumstances is recommended because alcohols, chlorhexidine, iodophors, and other antiseptic agents have poor activity against spores (II) (*120,172,224,225*).

- No recommendation can be made regarding the routine use of non-alcohol-based hand rubs for hand hygiene in health-care settings. Unresolved issue.

Figure 10.2 — CDC Hand-Hygiene Recommendations (cont.)

2. Hand-hygiene technique

- When decontaminating hands with an alcohol-based hand rub, apply product to palm of one hand and rub hands together, covering all surfaces of hands and fingers, until hands are dry (IB) (*288,410*). Follow the manufacturer's recommendations regarding the volume of product to use.

- When washing hands with soap and water, wet hands first with water, apply an amount of product recommended by the manufacturer to hands, and rub hands together vigorously for at least 15 seconds, covering all surfaces of the hands and fingers. Rinse hands with water and dry thoroughly with a disposable towel. Use towel to turn off the faucet (IB) (*90-92,94,411*). Avoid using hot water, because repeated exposure to hot water may increase the risk of dermatitis (IB) (*254,255*).

- Liquid, bar, leaflet or powdered forms of plain soap are acceptable when washing hands with a non-antimicrobial soap and water. When bar soap is used, soap racks that facilitate drainage and small bars of soap should be used (II) (*412-415*).

- Multiple-use cloth towels of the hanging or roll type are not recommended for use in healthcare settings (II) (*137,300*).

3. Surgical hand antisepsis

- Remove rings, watches, and bracelets before beginning the surgical hand scrub (II) (*375,378,416*).

- Remove debris from underneath fingernails using a nail cleaner under running water (II) (*14,417*).

- Surgical hand antisepsis using either an antimicrobial soap or an alcohol-based hand rub with persistent activity is recommended before donning sterile gloves when performing surgical procedures (IB) (*115,159,232,234,237,418*).

- When performing surgical hand antisepsis using an antimicrobial soap, scrub hands and forearms for the length of time recommended by the manufacturer, usually 2–6 minutes. Long scrub times (e.g., 10 minutes) are not necessary (IB) (*117,156,205, 207,238-241*).

- When using an alcohol-based surgical hand-scrub product with persistent activity, follow the manufacturer's instructions. Before applying the alcohol solution, prewash hands and forearms with a non-antimicrobial soap and dry hands and forearms completely. After application of the alcohol-based product as recommended, allow hands and forearms to dry thoroughly before donning sterile gloves (IB) (*159,237*).

4. Selection of hand-hygiene agents

- Provide personnel with efficacious hand-hygiene products that have low irritancy potential, particularly when these products are used multiple times per shift (IB) (*90,92,98,166,249*). This

> **Figure 10.2** **CDC HAND-HYGIENE RECOMMENDATIONS (CONT.)**
>
> recommendation applies to products used for hand antisepsis before and after patient care in clinical areas and to products used for surgical hand antisepsis by surgical personnel.
>
> - To maximize acceptance of hand-hygiene products by HCWs, solicit input from these employees regarding the feel, fragrance, and skin tolerance of any products under consideration. The cost of hand-hygiene products should not be the primary factor influencing product selection (IB) (*92,93,166, 274,276-278*).
>
> - When selecting non-antimicrobial soaps, antimicrobial soaps, or alcohol-based hand rubs, solicit information from manufacturers regarding any known interactions between products used to clean hands, skin care products, and the types of gloves used in the institution (II) (*174,372*).
>
> - Before making purchasing decisions, evaluate the dispenser systems of various product manufacturers or distributors to ensure that dispensers function adequately and deliver an appropriate volume of product (II) (*286*).
>
> - Do not add soap to a partially empty soap dispenser. This practice of "topping off" dispensers can lead to bacterial contamination of soap (IA) (*187,419*).
>
> **5. Skin care**
>
> - Provide HCWs with hand lotions or creams to minimize the occurrence of irritant contact dermatitis associated with hand antisepsis or handwashing (IA) (*272,273*).
>
> - Solicit information from manufacturers regarding any effects that hand lotions, creams, or alcohol-based hand antiseptics may have on the persistent effects of antimicrobial soaps being used in the institution (IB) (*174,420,421*).
>
> **6. Other aspects of hand hygiene**
>
> - Do not wear artificial fingernails or extenders when having direct contact with patients at high risk (e.g., those in intensive-care units or operating rooms) (IA) (*350—353*).
>
> - Keep natural nails tips less than 1/4-inch long (II) (*350*).
>
> - Wear gloves when contact with blood or other potentially infectious materials, mucous membranes, and nonintact skin could occur (IC) (*356*).
>
> - Remove gloves after caring for a patient. Do not wear the same pair of gloves for the care of more than one patient, and do not wash gloves between uses with different patients (IB) (*50,58,321,373*).
>
> - Change gloves during patient care if moving from a contaminated body site to a clean body site (II) (*50,51,58*).
>
> - No recommendation can be made regarding wearing rings in health-care settings. Unresolved issue.

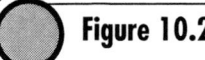

Figure 10.2 — **CDC HAND-HYGIENE RECOMMENDATIONS (CONT.)**

7. Health-care worker educational and motivational programs

- As part of an overall program to improve hand-hygiene practices of HCWs, educate personnel regarding the types of patient-care activities that can result in hand contamination and the advantages and disadvantages of various methods used to clean their hands (II) (*74,292,295,299*).

- Monitor HCWs' adherence with recommended hand-hygiene practices and provide personnel with information regarding their performance (IA) (*74,276,292,295,299,306,310*).

- Encourage patients and their families to remind HCWs to decontaminate their hands (II) (*394,422*).

8. Administrative measures

- Make improved hand-hygiene adherence an institutional priority and provide appropriate administrative support and financial resources (IB) (*74,75*).

- Implement a multidisciplinary program designed to improve adherence of health personnel to recommended hand-hygiene practices (IB) (*74,75*).

- As part of a multidisciplinary program to improve hand-hygiene adherence, provide HCWs with a readily accessible alcohol-based hand-rub product (IA) (*74,166,283,294,312*).

- To improve hand-hygiene adherence among personnel who work in areas in which high workloads and high intensity of patient care are anticipated, make an alcohol-based hand rub available at the entrance to the patient's room or at the bedside, in other convenient locations, and in individual pocket-sized containers to be carried by HCWs (IA) (*11,74,166,283,284,312,318,423*).

- Store supplies of alcohol-based hand rubs in cabinets or areas approved for flammable materials (IC).

Part III. Performance indicators

1. The following performance indicators are recommended for measuring improvements in HCWs' hand-hygiene adherence:

    H. Periodically monitor and record adherence as the number of hand-hygiene episodes performed by personnel/number of hand-hygiene opportunities, by ward or by service. Provide feedback to personnel regarding their performance.

- Monitor the volume of alcohol-based hand rub (or detergent used for handwashing or hand antisepsis) used per 1,000 patient-days.

- Monitor adherence to policies dealing with wearing of artificial nails.

- When outbreaks of infection occur, assess the adequacy of health-care worker hand hygiene.

HAND-HYGIENE SAFETY GOAL

Figure 10.3

HAND-HYGIENE OBSERVATION TOOL

Date of Observation _____   Location _____   Time Observed _____

Professional Observed	Compliance	Noncompliance	Noncompliant Act (i.e. no hand hygiene before patient contact, handwashing too short, etc.)	Bed #	Observation Description (i.e. procedure, type of contact, gloves, etc.)
☐ RN ☐ PCT ☐ MD ☐ RT ☐ Other_____	☐ HW ☐ Foam ☐ Other Time:_____	☐ HW ☐ Foam ☐ Other Time:_____			
☐ RN ☐ PCT ☐ MD ☐ RT ☐ Other_____	☐ HW ☐ Foam ☐ Other Time:_____	☐ HW ☐ Foam ☐ Other Time:_____			
☐ RN ☐ PCT ☐ MD ☐ RT ☐ Other_____	☐ HW ☐ Foam ☐ Other Time:_____	☐ HW ☐ Foam ☐ Other Time:_____			
☐ RN ☐ PCT ☐ MD ☐ RT ☐ Other_____	☐ HW ☐ Foam ☐ Other Time:_____	☐ HW ☐ Foam ☐ Other Time:_____			
☐ RN ☐ PCT ☐ MD ☐ RT ☐ Other_____	☐ HW ☐ Foam ☐ Other Time:_____	☐ HW ☐ Foam ☐ Other Time:_____			
☐ RN ☐ PCT ☐ MD ☐ RT ☐ Other_____	☐ HW ☐ Foam ☐ Other Time:_____	☐ HW ☐ Foam ☐ Other Time:_____			
☐ RN ☐ PCT ☐ MD ☐ RT ☐ Other_____	☐ HW ☐ Foam ☐ Other Time:_____	☐ HW ☐ Foam ☐ Other Time:_____			
☐ RN ☐ PCT ☐ MD ☐ RT ☐ Other_____	☐ HW ☐ Foam ☐ Other Time:_____	☐ HW ☐ Foam ☐ Other Time:_____			
☐ RN ☐ PCT ☐ MD ☐ RT ☐ Other_____	☐ HW ☐ Foam ☐ Other Time:_____	☐ HW ☐ Foam ☐ Other Time:_____			

RN or LPN – royal blue or white
MD – lab coat or sea green surgical scrubs
RT – green PCT – navy or light blue CT/PT - aqua

Observer: _____

Printed with permission from the Center for Infectious Diseases, Memorial Health University Medical Center, Savannah, GA.

CHAPTER TEN

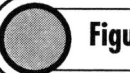

Figure 10.4 — CDC HAND-HYGIENE GUIDELINES FACT SHEET

- Improved adherence to hand hygiene (i.e. hand washing or use of alcohol-based hand rubs) has been shown to terminate outbreaks in health care facilities, to reduce transmission of antimicrobial resistant organisms (e.g. methicillin resistant staphylococcus aureus) and reduce overall infection rates.

- CDC is releasing guidelines to improve adherence to hand hygiene in health care settings. In addition to traditional handwashing with soap and water, CDC is recommending the use of alcohol-based handrubs by health care personnel for patient care because they address some of the obstacles that health care professionals face when taking care of patients.

- Handwashing with soap and water remains a sensible strategy for hand hygiene in non-health care settings and is recommended by CDC and other experts.

- When health care personnel's hands are visibly soiled, they should wash with soap and water.

- The use of gloves does not eliminate the need for hand hygiene. Likewise, the use of hand hygiene does not eliminate the need for gloves. Gloves reduce hand contamination by 70 percent to 80 percent, prevent cross-contamination and protect patients and health care personnel from infection. Handrubs should be used before and after each patient just as gloves should be changed before and after each patient.

- When using an alcohol-based handrub, apply product to palm of one hand and rub hands together, covering all surfaces of hands and fingers, until hands are dry. Note that the volume needed to reduce the number of bacteria on hands varies by product.

- Alcohol-based handrubs significantly reduce the number of microorganisms on skin, are fast acting and cause less skin irritation.

- Health care personnel should avoid wearing artificial nails and keep natural nails less than one quarter of an inch long if they care for patients at high risk of acquiring infections (e.g. patients in intensive care units or in transplant units.

- When evaluating hand hygiene products for potential use in health care facilities, administrators or product selection committees should consider the relative efficacy of antiseptic agents against various pathogens and the acceptability of hand hygiene products by personnel. Characteristics of a product that can affect acceptance and therefore usage include its smell, consistency, color and the effect of dryness on hands.

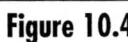

Figure 10.4 CDC HAND-HYGIENE GUIDELINES FACT SHEET (CONT.)

- As part of these recommendations, CDC is asking health care facilities to develop and implement a system for measuring improvements in adherence to these hand hygiene recommendations. Some of the suggested performance indicators include: periodic monitoring of hand hygiene adherence and providing feedback to personnel regarding their performance, monitoring the volume of alcohol-based handrub used/1000 patient days, monitoring adherence to policies dealing with wearing artificial nails and focused assessment of the adequacy of health care personnel hand hygiene when outbreaks of infection occur.

- Allergic contact dermatitis due to alcohol hand rubs is very uncommon. However, with increasing use of such products by health care personnel, it is likely that true allergic reactions to such products will occasionally be encountered.

- Alcohol-based hand rubs take less time to use than traditional hand washing. In an eight-hour shift, an estimated one hour of an ICU nurse's time will be saved by using an alcohol-based handrub.

- These guidelines should not be construed to legalize product claims that are not allowed by an FDA product approval by FDA's Over-the-Counter Drug Review. The recommendations are not intended to apply to consumer use of the products discussed.

Fact sheet available at *www.cdc.gov/od/oc/media/pressrel/fs021025.*

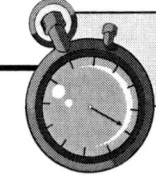

Figure 10.5 — Hand-Hygiene Policy

PURPOSE:

To decrease the risk of transmission of infection by appropriate hand hygiene.

POLICY:

Hand hygiene is generally considered the single most important procedure for preventing healthcare-associated infections. Antiseptics control or kill microorganisms contaminating skin and other superficial tissues and are sometimes composed of the same chemicals that are used for disinfection of inanimate objects. Although antiseptics and other hand-hygiene agents do not sterilize the skin, they can reduce microbial contamination depending on the type and the amount of contamination, the agent used, the presence of residual activity, and the hand-hygiene technique followed.

I. HAND HYGIENE

When hands are visibly dirty or contaminated with proteinaceous material or are visibly soiled with blood or other body fluids, wash hands with either a non-antimicrobial soap and water or an antimicrobial soap and water.

A. Turn on water to a comfortable warm temperature.

B. Moisten hands with soap and water and make a heavy lather.

C. Wash well under running water for a minimum of 15 seconds, using a rotary motion and friction.

D. Rinse hands well under running water.

E. Turn off faucet with paper towel and discard.

F. Dry hands with a clean paper towel and discard.

II. WATERLESS HAND-HYGIENE PRODUCTS

If hands are not visibly soiled, use an alcohol-based hand rub for routinely decontaminating hands in all clinical situations other than those listed under "hand hygiene" above.

A. When decontaminating hands with an alcohol-based hand rub, apply product to palm of one hand and rub hands together, covering all surfaces of hands and fingers, until hands are dry.

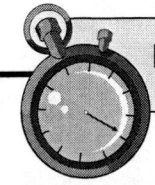

Figure 10.5 — HAND-HYGIENE POLICY (CONT.)

B. Follow the manufacturer's recommendations regarding the volume of product to use.

C. Waterless handwash stations should be strategically placed to be used as an adjunct to soap and water handwash. Note: Flammability of product is an issue. Check with state and local fire guidelines before placement and bulk storage.

III. HAND LOTIONS

The healthcare facility may choose to provide a hand lotion—approved by the Infection Control Committee—that is compatible for use with hand hygiene products and gloves already in use by facility.

Note: Some products interfere with persistence of skin antiseptics or glove integrity.

- Hand-lotion stations should be installed near handwash stations.

- Hand lotions should not be allowed to be brought from home. Contaminated hand lotions have been implicated in outbreaks of diseases (primarily gram negative rods) in healthcare facilities. Large bottles or poorly designed nozzles can become colonized, allowing for spread of microorganisms on the hands of healthcare workers.

Source: HCPro, Infection Control Manual for Hospitals, 2004

Chapter Eleven

Sentinel event safety goal

Safety goal

This chapter addresses the Joint Commission on Accreditation of Healthcare Organizations (JCAHO) National Patient Safety Goal #7b, which requires facilities to manage specific healthcare-acquired infections (HAI) as sentinel events.

> **How to survey the goal:**
> - Interview leaders
> - Interview infection control (IC) staff
>
> **Documents that may be requested or reviewed:**
> - Minutes of the IC committee
> - Documentation of sentinel events and root-cause analysis (RCA)

> **Safety Goal #7:** Reduce the risk of healthcare-acquired infections.
> **Safety goal #7b:** Manage as sentinel events all identified cases of unanticipated death or major permanent loss of function associated with a healthcare-associated infection.

Goal #7b has proven problematic for IC programs across the nation. The main concern of infection control professionals (ICP) is determining which cases of patients who die and have HAIs should be managed as sentinel events, since many patients who die with an HAI are very sick and have multiple other problems. The JCAHO has responded to ICPs' concerns this way:

> "This determination is based on the condition of the patient at the time of admission to the organization. A death or major permanent loss of function should be considered a sentinel event if the outcome was not the result of the natural course of the patient's illness or underlying condition(s) that existed at the time of admission. For example, an otherwise healthy patient who is admitted for an elective procedure, develops a wound infection, becomes septic, and dies should be considered a sentinel event. However, cases in which the patient is immunocompromised or elderly with multiple co-morbidities are more difficult to classify. The knowledge that a certain percentage of patients with a given condition will die does not mean that the death of any one of these patients is "anticipated." If, at the time of admission, the patient's condition is such that he or she has a high likelihood of not surviving the episode of care (e.g., the hospitalization), then that patient's death would not be considered a sentinel event. Otherwise, it should be managed as a sentinel event, that is, a root-cause analysis should be conducted."
> (http://www.jcaho.org/accredited+organizations/patient+safety04+npsg/index.html#goal7.)

ICPs have voiced concerns about both the amount of time required to identify cases considered sentinel events and how long it will take to conduct root-cause analyses (RCA). The JCAHO has responded that it does not expect hospitals to undergo increased or otherwise modified surveillance activities. It further states that ICP participation on the RCA team could be very beneficial—and most ICPs likely would concur with the JCAHO since they have knowledge of infection prevention and control activities that could prevent future infections from becoming sentinel events.

Many IC programs, prior to safety goal #7b, did not have methods in place for reviewing deaths to determine whether the patient had an HAI and whether the death qualified as a sentinel event. Therefore, the workloads of many IC programs have increased with this new standard.

The best scenario for such IC programs is to use the skills of the person who manages the sentinel event/RCA process by having him or her notify the IC department when a potential sentinel event involving an HAI is being reviewed. The ICP then could get involved with the review team to determine whether the event actually qualifies as a sentinel event, to identify the root causes, and to take preventive measures to prevent future occurrences of such an event.

Once your facility identifies an HAI sentinel event, conduct a credible RCA within 45 days of the event. The RCA will prompt healthcare staff to ask the question "why did this happen" repeatedly, for each step in the sentinel event, until they can determine the root cause. Only after determining the root cause can healthcare staff take appropriate interventions to prevent a similar occurrence. A credible RCA should be thorough and should identify system and process factors that may be redesigned to reduce the risk of serious adverse patient outcomes.

ICPs involved with the Association for Professionals in Infection Control and Epidemiology (APIC) have developed excellent information on sentinel events and methods of completing an RCA specific to IC (see Figures 11.1–11.4 for examples. The documents are titled "Integrating Sentinel Event Analysis into Your Infection Contro Practice," January 2004.)

- Figure 11.1 answers questions specifically relating to sentinel events and RCAs involving IC
- Figure 11.2 enhances the basic RCA format to make it specific to IC
- Figure 11.3 lists 21 steps in preparing for an RCA using the format of FOCUS-PDCA
- Figure 11.4 provides three scenarios that demonstrate potential HAI sentinel events

Figures 11.1-11.4 are used with permission from APIC and may be found at www.apic.org under the "patient safety" link.

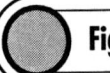

Figure 11.1 — SENTINAL EVENTS AND RCAs

Developers: Janet Frain, Denise Murphy, Georgia Dash, and Marie Kassai
January 2004

What is a sentinel event?

The JCAHO defines a sentinel event as "an unexpected occurrence involving death or serious physical or psychological injury." Serious injury specifically includes loss of limb or function. The JCAHO further prescribes a list of "reviewable" sentinel events as

- unexpected deaths
- unanticipated major loss of function
- infant abduction
- infant discharged to wrong family
- rape
- hemolytic transfusion reaction
- surgery on the wrong patient or body part
- patient suicide

The facility can certainly determine other types of events for which a root-cause analysis (RCA) is an appropriate investigative and problem-resolution tool.

What is the relevance to your practice as an ICP?

ICPs actively involved in surveillance activities would most likely identify unexpected deaths or unanticipated major loss of function due to infection as a potential sentinel event. Some of these cases are clearly identifiable but, unfortunately, many are not. Each case has to be evaluated individually. Use the help of your internal resources to make this determination. The requirement to do RCAs has been in place for four years now. Each facility has a department or person who is responsible for "managing" this process. Use that person, an Infectious Diseases expert, your Administrator, and Medical Staff leadership to work with you to identify these cases.

What skills do I have to contribute to this process?

The ICP is an extremely valuable member of the patient care team. Your experience with outbreak management and ability to identify infectious events, evaluate likely sources for infection, recognize standards that help prevent transmission or development of an infection, and analyze medical literature make you an excellent resource to the team.

Chapter Eleven

Figure 11.1 — **Sentinal Events and RCAs (cont.)**

What happens once the ICP identifies a sentinel event?

A credible root-cause analysis has to be completed within 45 days of the event occurring. The Joint Commission has created a framework to use to make sure all elements are addressed (Attachment A). The team should tackle each of these content areas to help identify contributing factors, identify root cause, and put effective control measures in place to reduce the risk of recurrence.

How does a root-cause analysis differ from an epidemiologic investigation?

Denise Murphy has created an excellent crosswalk for a comparison of the two methodologies (Attachment B). There are many similarities in the two processes. A root-cause analysis focuses on individual events based on patient outcome. The process we use to investigate an epidemiologic investigation typically looks at clusters of infections or individual cases of epidemiologic importance. It is not dependent on patient outcome.

What is my job in a root-cause analysis?

The ICP can participate either as the team leader or a team member. If the ICP accepts the role of Team Leader, it is important to remember that you are there primarily as a content expert. Carefully listening as participants describe the processes leading to the untoward event is an important skill. You know what the Infection Control standards are; therefore, you are the person most qualified to identify gaps or compliance issues.

Other team members would include front-line staff most involved in the process, an Infectious Diseases physician, and other appropriate members of the medical staff. It's important to remember that these may be very emotionally charged meetings, so the ICP as a Team Leader should know techniques for "de-fusing" sensitive situations.

Warning: It is not unusual for clinicians to debate the clinical management or specific aspects of the case. For example, did the patient die from the infection or was the cardiac status so fragile that the patient would have expired anyway? While this level of review is important, the peer review committee may be the more appropriate setting for a decision. The root-cause analysis focuses on systems and processes. The Team Leader and/or facilitator must skillfully bring the group back to this focus.

In addition, it is important that the message be delivered very early on in the meeting that ALL participants are on equal footing and everyone should contribute. For many groups, this will be the first time physicians and staff have actually sat in the same room to analyze an event.

What does success look like?

A credible and successful RCA identifies all the elements that contributed to an event, develops action plans to prevent recurrence and ensures that those actions are completed. A very important component of a RCA is thorough review of the literature to ensure that action plans are based on best practices and appropriate standards.

As labor-intensive as an RCA is, it is never a waste of time!

Figure 11.2 — ENHANCING THE RCA FORMAT

Developers: Janet Frain, Denise Murphy, Georgia Dash and Marie Kassai
January 2004

Attachment A

Level of Analysis		Questions	Findings
What happened?	Sentinel Event	What are the details of the event? (Brief description)	What type of infection did the patient have that caused the death or permanent loss of function?
		When did the event occur? (Date, day of week, time)	
		What area/service was impacted?	Surgery? ICU? Pulmonary Services? Transplant unit?
Why did it happen?	The process or activity in which the event occurred.	What are the steps in the process, as designed? (A flow diagram may be helpful here)	Sterilization process? Skin preparation process? Prophylactic antibiotic administration? Environmental cleaning? **The process should be flowcharted "as is," so critical steps can be identified.**
What were the most proximate factors?		What steps were involved in (contributed to) the event?	Were instruments cleaned adequately before putting in the sterilizer? Was the cycle allowed to complete? Was the skin prep rushed because everyone was in a hurry to start the case? Was the abx given at the right time pre-op (or at all?)? **Analyze the flowchart and determine the gaps.**
(Typically "special cause" variation)	Human factors	What human factors were relevant to the outcome?	Did staff feel pressured to get the job done quickly? Were critical steps missed because they thought they weren't important? Have shortcuts been built into the system? **Participants have to be painfully honest without fear of retribution!**
	Equipment factors	How did the equipment performance affect the outcome?	Was the appropriate preventive maintenance done? Was the staff oriented appropriately to equipment? Types of equipment may be autoclaves, sterilizers, ventilators, all types of tubing's connected to the patient, etc
	Controllable environmental factors	What factors directly affected the outcome?	Was the staff in a hurry? Is clean equipment stored near contaminated equipment? Does the staff have what they need when they need it? Were there distractions that interrupted the process? **Is the area they are working in conducive to the process?**
	Uncontrollable external factors	Are they truly beyond the organization's control?	Are there productivity standards for MDs that force them to hurry through processes?

Figure 11.2 — Enhancing the RCA Format (cont.)

Level of Analysis		Questions	Findings
Why did that happen? What systems and processes underlie those proximate factors? (Common cause variation here may lead to special cause variation in dependent processes)	Other	Are there any other factors that have directly influenced this outcome?	This is the time for the group to brainstorm other systems or processes that they feel contributed to the outcome
		What other areas or services are impacted	
	Human Resources issues	To what degree is staff properly qualified and currently competent for their responsibilities?	Is the right skill level person performing the function? Is orientation adequate? Have the staff demonstrated competency on the equipment they are using? Has competency with the process been demonstrated? Are the learning needs of the individual taken into consideration when training/orienting new employees? This is the time to ask all relevant questions about adequate education and training for the process.
		How did actual staffing compare with ideal levels?	Was the department running short that day? Did the therapists have time to do their rounds? Were tubing changes let go due to inadequate staff? Are there enough people to do the job? Ideal staffing levels are difficult to determine. Comparison with industry standards, if available, can be helpful.
		What are the plans for dealing with contingencies that would tend to reduce effective staffing levels?	What does the department do if they are "short-staffed" for the day? Who prioritizes? What realistic options for replacement personnel are available to the manager?
		To what degree is staff performance in the operant process(es) addressed?	How do we know the staff is competent to do the procedure? Is there adequate supervision? Are the staff allowed to find creative shortcuts? Does staff understand their role in reducing infectious complications as part of the process they work in?
		How can orientation and in-service training be improved?	Brainstorm and listen carefully to the front-line caregiver that knows best what will and will not work. Once an event of this nature occurs, staff really think about their role and what could be done better. They don't want a repeat incident!
	Information management issues	To what degree is all necessary information available when needed? Accurate? Complete? Unambiguous?	Are there procedures available to the staff? What information about the patient was passed on in report? Any critical information omitted? Did the therapist know they had to see the patient? Is the procedure for sterile dressing changes complete? Did the pre-op nurse know the pre-op antibiotic had not been given? This information can be found in documents, on-line, direct communications, shift reports, etc

Figure 11.2 — Enhancing the RCA Format (cont.)

Level of Analysis	Questions	Findings
	To what degree is communication among participants adequate?	Was the technician comfortable telling the physician that the skin prep was not complete? That the equipment had been rushed through the sterilization process? **This is a critical question when doing a root cause analysis — communication breakdown has been the root cause in many events**
Environmental management issues	To what degree was the physical environment appropriate for the processes being carried out?	Is the staff member able to work uninterrupted? Is the sink placed in such a way that it makes hand washing cumbersome? Are fans blowing through dirty work areas? Is the ventilator equipment stored appropriately? Are the surgical supplies in a clean, dry area, away from contamination? **This sometimes requires a site visit by the team to the area in question.**
	What systems are in place to identify environmental risks?	**Does the hospital have a process for content experts to make assessments of environmental risks? Is the ICP a welcome visitor in Surgery? Are the issues identified acted upon and is there accountability?**
	What emergency and failure-mode responses have been planned and tested?	The group can brainstorm all potential failure modes associated with the process and determine what interventions would be most helpful to prevent that potential failure mode? This is a very labor-intensive process.
Leadership issues: - Corporate culture	To what degree is the culture conducive to risk identification and reduction?	Is the staff comfortable in reporting risks? Is their manager responsive? Does the staff know what to do if no action is taken? **Asking this question may reveal some serious systems issues or management issues that leadership should be aware of and must act on.**
- Encouragement of communication	What are the barriers to communication of potential risk factors?	Is the manager available to the staff? Are all opinions respected, regardless of skill level? **Processes may need to be developed to allow free and open communication**
- Clear communication of priorities	To what degree is the prevention of adverse outcomes communicated as a high priority? How?	Has the staff been educated on patient safety and prevention of adverse outcomes? Do they understand the rationale for each step in a process to reduce risk of infectious outcomes? Does the Environmental Services employee understand how critical their role is in infection prevention and control? **How is the department-specific orientation to infection prevention and control communicated to the staff?**
Uncontrollable factors	What can be done to protect against the effects of these uncontrollable factors?	Brainstorm with the group.

- For each of the findings identified in the analysis as needing an action, indicate the planned action expected, implementation date and associated measure of effectiveness.
- If after consideration of such a finding, a decision is made not to implement an associated risk reduction strategy, indicate the rationale for not taking action at this time. OR...
- Check to be sure that the selected measure will provide data that will permit assessment of the effectiveness of the action.
- Consider whether pilot testing of a planned improvement should be conducted.
- Improvements to reduce risk should ultimately be implemented in all areas where applicable, not just where the event occurred. Identify where the improvements will be implemented.

Figure 11.3 — APIC Comparison of RCA and Outbreak Investigation

FOCUS-PDCA	Steps in Preparing for a Root Cause Analysis		Outbreak Investigation
Find An Opportunity			
Organize a Team	Step 1	Organize a Team	1. Confirm existence of outbreak
Clarify the Current Process	Step 2	Define the Problem	2. Confirm diagnosis of cases
	Step 3	Study the Problem	3. Prepare or investigation
Understand Variation	Step 4	Determine What Happened	4. Create case definition
	Step 5	Identify Contributing Process Factors	5. Search for additional cases
	Step 6	Identify Other Contributing Factors	6. Characterize epidemic by person, place, time (line list)
	Step 7	Measure – Collect and Assess Data on Proximate and Underlying Causes	7. Generate tentative hypothesis
	Step 8	Design and Implement Interim Changes	8. Test hypothesis
	Step 9	Identify Which Systems Are Involved – Root Causes	9. Institute additional studies
	Step 10	Prune the List of Root Causes	10. Iimplement interventions
	Step 11	Confirm Root Causes	11. Communicate findings
Select the improvement solution	Step 12	Explore and Identify Risk Reduction Strategies	12. Move to process improvement!
Plan the Improvement	Step 13	Formulate Improvement Actions	
	Step 14	Evaluate Proposed Improvement Actions	
	Step 15	Design Improvements	
	Step 16	Ensure Acceptability of the Action Plan	
Do the Improvement and Collect Data	Step 17	Implement the Improvement Plan	
Check and Study the Results	Step 18	Develop Measures of Effectiveness and Ensure Their Success	
	Step 19	Evaluate Implementation of Improvement Efforts	
Act and Hold the Gain	Step 20	Take Additional Action	
	Step 21	Communicate the Results	

(PLAN – DO – CHECK – ACT cycle)

Figure 11.4 — HAI Sentinel Events

Developers: Janet Frain, Denise Murphy, Georgia Dash, and Marie Kassai, January 2004

SCENARIO ONE

A 73-year-old male was admitted with aortic stenosis. The patient also had diabetes mellitus. He underwent an aortic valve replacement. He had an uneventful recovery and was ready for discharge nine days post-op.

On the day of discharge, the staff RN was removing the saline lock from the right forearm. The nurse noticed a small, reddened area around the site. The nurse reported the findings to the physician, who ordered wet soaks, but did not delay the discharge. The patient's temperature was 99.4°F. This was not reported to the physician.

Twenty-four hours after discharge, the patient was readmitted with a temperature of 103°F and was acutely ill. Cultures from the saline lock site, spinal fluid, blood, urine, and sputum were all positive for Staph aureus. The patient expired.

Would this be considered a sentinel event?

While the risk of any operative procedure certainly includes infection, this patient's infection and death were most likely not related to his surgical procedure. He had a very normal post-operative course. There appeared to be an infection starting at his IV site that was left untreated. While we cannot say with 100% certainty that the true source of infection was the IV site, it did appear this was the proximate cause of his ultimate demise.

A root-cause analysis in this unexpected death would analyze several systems issues:
- What is the policy for changing saline locks? What are the assessment expectations if the saline lock is not changed?
- Does this nursing unit have a policy that all patients on their unit will have a saline lock, regardless of the patient condition?
- Were the nurses doing the assessment competent in assessment and maintenance of IV saline locks?
- Was the appropriate information communicated to the physician?
- Were the staffing levels appropriate for the needs of the patients on this unit? Did the nurses feel rushed to discharge a patient?
- Were there other factors that could have potentially diverted the nurse from conveying all necessary information to the physician prior to discharge?
- Should the physician have delayed discharge? Were there external factors influencing the surgeon's decision to discharge (monitoring of LOS by the MD group for example)?

Typically, several systems issues will be identified that will result in a plan of action. In this case, it may be policy and procedures changes, staff competency assessment, and peer review.

Figure 11.4 — HAI Sentinel Events (cont.)

SCENARIO TWO

A 24-year-old mother underwent a c/section for fetal distress at 32 weeks. The infant weighed 4 lbs 3 oz. at birth but appeared to be in no acute distress. The infant was admitted to the Neonatal ICU for close observation. The infant progressed well and did not require intubation, intravenous lines or any invasive procedures.

As is the policy in this facility, Mom was instructed to pump her breasts for feedings. Mom used the new electronic breast pump that was stored at the nurse's station on the Post Partum unit. Mom elected to go home without her baby on day four to care for her other children at home. When she came back to the hospital, she continued to use the breast pump from Post Partum.

The infant gained weight and was scheduled for discharge. The evening before discharge, the infant became irritable and had episodes of bradycardia. The neonatologist on call immediately ordered blood cultures and empiric antibiotics. The blood cultures were positive for *Pseudomonas aeruginosa*. Despite aggressive therapy by the physicians, the baby expired.

Would this be considered a sentinel event?

This infant, while certainly pre-term, experienced a very uneventful hospital stay. While the infant was housed in the NICU, he did not have any of the invasive procedures that the ICP would normally associate with a stay in that unit. The infant was scheduled for discharge and had an abrupt change in condition that resulted in death.

A root-cause analysis in this unexpected death would analyze several systems issues:
- What is the policy for cleaning and storing the electronic breast pumps?
- Did the mother receive any education on hand hygiene, cleaning her breasts prior to pumping, and ascertaining that the breast pump was clean?
- Was the nurse competent in maternal-child care, including instruction for breast-feeding?
- The pump was new – was everyone on the unit oriented to that pump and how to use it?
- How was the breast milk stored?
- What education had the staff nurses in the NICU received on hand hygiene?
- What was the census in the NICU? Was there adequate staffing?
- Were there adequate safeguards in place to make sure the infant got the correct mother's milk?

The risk in this setting would be to only focus on the issue of the breast pump. Experienced ICPs realize that many factors could have contributed to this infection. Continually asking, "Why," will ultimately get to the root-cause.

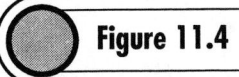

HAI SENTINEL EVENTS (CONT.)

SCENARIO THREE

A nine-year-old child is admitted to the Pediatric Unit with acute lymphocytic leukemia. This is a new diagnosis for this patient. She undergoes six weeks of chemotherapy in the hospital. As a result, her immune system was extremely compromised. She was kept in an isolation room for the last three weeks of her therapy as her white count had dropped to very low levels.

During week six in the hospital, the child spikes a fever to 104°F and is tachycardic. She complains of a new onset of pain in her head. This is reported to the Oncologist immediately and cultures are obtained from the blood, nasopharynx, and spinal tap. The spinal tap and the NP culture grow *Aspergillus fumigatus*. Despite aggressive treatment, the child eventually is taketo the operating room and has to have her left eye and cheekbone removed to prevent further damage from the *Aspergillus*. She is ultimately discharged home.

Would this be considered a sentinel event?

Some ICPs would argue that infections of this nature are a rare but well-known complication of this diagnosis and treatment regimen. This could be considered permanent loss of function. Many safeguards were probably put in place to prevent this tragic outcome. This event would warrant intense analysis at a minimum.

An intense analysis (or perhaps root-cause analysis) could analyze several systems issues:
- What engineering controls are in place to prevent acquisition of *Aspergillus*? Were the engineers adequately oriented and trained in the role of environmental pathogens for this patient population?
- What education and training did the nurses receive for this high-risk patient population?
- How are new employees oriented?
- What is the staffing ratio for these children? Do the assignments require nurses or other members of the healthcare team to care for children with infection as well as these immune suppressed children?
- What equipment was involved in the care of this patient? Any system breakdowns in cleaning processes?
- Is the medical staff working with these patients educated on appropriate barrier precautions and hand hygiene?
- Was there any construction going on in or around the facility?
- Were the parents taught about hand hygiene?

Because the ICP comes armed with the knowledge of microorganisms and how they are introduced or spread, the ICP's knowledge will be invaluable in reviewing the systems issues associated with this type of event.

CHAPTER TWELVE

Other standards related to IC

The overlap between the IC standards and standards within multiple other functions is great. The more functions in which a standard can be scored, the greater the weight of the standard. For example, if a JCAHO surveyor determines that staff are not appropriately oriented to IC, surveyors could cite requirements for improvement in IC, HR, and leadership. Be aware of the standards with overlap of functions so that any improvement in those standards becomes high priority.

This chapter provides information on standards outside the IC function that could impact IC and that are reflected in the JCAHO IC survey. Such standards may be found in human resources (HR), leadership, performance improvement (PI), and environment of care (EC).

Human resources

The primary standards for competency and qualifications of staff fall under HR. Although the IC standards address these issues in the IC department, surveyors may cite requirements for improvement in those areas in HR as well.

The JCAHO's HR survey will likely focus on the areas of competency and qualifications—including those related to IC—of all staff. Because IC staff are very involved in developing IC policies and practices throughout the facility, they play a vital collaborative role in determining which IC competencies staff in all departments need.

The HR standards require that you orient and train staff on the following:
- Policies and procedures
- Specific job duties and responsibilities relating to IC
- Risks within the hospital environment, including risk of exposure to infectious diseases
- Actions to eliminate, minimize, or report risks

- Procedures to follow in the event of an incident
- Reporting processes

Then, in your ongoing inservices, training, or other activities, emphasize job-related aspects of safety and IC. The OSHA bloodborne pathogens regulations require that staff in all departments know the specific IC and safety risks they may encounter. For example, maintenance staff who work on air-handling systems in areas that house tuberculosis patients or emergency staff who encounter pediatric patients with undiagnosed airborne diseases must be informed of the situation's risks and precautions to take.

Leadership

The leadership standards require leaders to define the qualifications and competence of staff who provide care, treatment, and services, and to recommend a sufficient number of qualified, competent staff.

The leaders also must ensure that the hospital uses an integrated patient safety program, which, of course, includes the IC program. The IC standards also call for the leaders to assess the effectiveness of the IC program.

Environment of care

The EC standards do the following:

1. Require that a team of staff members conduct environmental tours to detect areas for improvements within multiple departments (e.g., maintenance, housekeeping, IC, etc). ICPs in many hospitals are part of these teams to help integrate IC—such as hand hygiene, sanitation, isolation, and use of personal protective equipment—into the elements reviewed on tour. See Figure 12.1 on page 106 for a sample environmental tour form for IC.

2. Address the management of hazardous materials and wastes. The written management plan should include handling, storage, disposal, and transport of biomedical waste.

3. Address having a written emergency management plan. This plan should address the IC requirement for a planned response to an influx, or risk of influx, of infectious patients.

4. Address demolition, construction, renovation, and the need for risk criteria that address, among

other things, IC. The Association for Professionals in Infection Control and Epidemiology offers an excellent book to assist ICPs plan for demolition, construction, and renovation activities: Infection Control During Construction and Renovations, 2nd Edition, 2002. An additional resource is the Centers for Disease Control and Prevention (CDC) Guidelines for "Environmental Infection Control in Healthcare Facilities: Recommendations of CDC and the Healthcare Infection Control Practice Advisory Committee" (HICPAC). MMWR 52 no. RR-10 (2003). Download it from the CDC Web site at www.cdc.gov/ncidod/hip/enviro/guide.htm. Figure 12.2 on page 110 includes CDC recommendations from the document listed above.

Performance improvement

The PI function relates directly to IC. The standards and elements of performance include collecting data, systematically aggregating and analyzing the data, analyzing undesirable trends in performance, identifying and managing sentinel events, using data analysis to improve performance, and reducing risks of sentinel events. All of these elements are components of the IC program and, as such, requirements for improvement for IC could be cited under PI as well.

Chapter Twelve

Figure 12.1 — **INFECTION CONTROL ROUNDS**

Area/Department:		Date of Review:		Reviewer:		
CRITERIA	**REQUIREMENTS**	**RATING**			**ACTION NEEDED:**	
		C	NI	N/A		
Patient rooms	Horizontal surfaces are clean					
	No visible soil on vertical surfaces					
	Trash cans not overflowing					
	Bathroom is clean					
	Hand hygiene products available					
	Soap and paper towels available					
	PPE available as needed					
Isolation rooms	Appropriate signage in place					
	Supplies and PPE available					
	Trash and linen handled per policy					
	Appropriate PPE used by staff					
	Appropriate patient/family education					
	Airborne precautions:					
	• Door closed					
	• Negative pressure is monitored					
	• Appropriate air exchanges					
Hand hygiene	Sinks for handwashing are appropriately stocked with soap, paper towels, trash cans					
	Sinks are available in all areas as needed					
	Alcohol handrubs are available in patients' rooms and other areas as needed					
	Placement of alcohol handrubs is compliant with safety recommendations					
	Handwashing/hand hygiene is monitored for staff compliance					
Refrigerators	Daily temperature checks are documented and appropriate temps maintained					
	Refrigerator has a single use (medication, foods, specimens)					
	Items are appropriately labeled					

C= compliance   NI= needs improvement   NA= not applicable

OTHER STANDARDS RELATED TO IC

Figure 12.1 — **INFECTION CONTROL ROUNDS (CONT.)**

CRITERIA	REQUIREMENTS	RATING C	NI	N/A	ACTION NEEDED:
	Refrigerator is clean and defrosted (if necessary)				
Linens (clean)	Linens are in good condition				
	Stored in covered cart or in linen room				
	Covered for transport				
Linens (soiled)	In hamper with impervious liner or hamper is cleaned on a specific schedule				
	Hamper is covered				
	Soiled linen covered for transport				
	Soiled linen is bagged at bedside				
	Removed from units/building on specified schedule				
Halls	Uncluttered				
	Horizontal and vertical surfaces are clean				
	No hallway obstruction				
	Full unobstructed access to exits				
Administrative areas: • Offices • Conference rooms • Nurses stations	Horizontal and vertical surfaces are clean				
	Trash is not overflowing				
	Carpet, if used, is not soiled				
	Bathrooms are clean				
Hazardous/ biohazard materials and biomedical waste	Storage areas have appropriate signage				
	OSHA compliant storage containers				
	Picked up for transport on specified schedule				
	Appropriate sharps containers in use				
	Sharps containers no more than 3/4 full				
	Sharps containers secured for transport				
	Appropriate biomedical waste manifests maintained				
Disinfection/ Sterilization	Equipment is in good working condition				

C= compliance   NI= needs improvement   NA= not applicable

Infection Control Compliance Guide: Understanding the JCAHO's Standards

Figure 12.1 — Infection Control Rounds (cont.)

CRITERIA	REQUIREMENTS	RATING C	NI	N/A	ACTION NEEDED:
	Appropriate processes in place for chemical disinfection				
	Appropriate sterilization records are maintained				
	Chemical/biological monitors are used as appropriate				
	Preventive maintenance program in place				
	Employee protection measures are implemented				
	Event-related sterilization packaging is used				
Storage	Storage areas are clean and uncluttered				
	Supplies are at least 18" from ceiling				
	Supplies are at least 6" from floor				
	Supplies are not stored under sinks				
Clean utility	Door to room is labeled				
	Environment is clean				
	Clean equipment is tagged/bagged as ready to use				
	No supplies stored under sink				
	All supplies off the floor				
Soiled utility	Door to room is labeled				
	Biohazard symbol on door if biomedical waste in room				
	Soiled linen in hamper with impervious liner or hamper is cleaned on specific schedule				
	Room is uncluttered				
	Clean supplies not in room				
	Appropriate PPE available				
Waiting areas	Horizontal and vertical surfaces are clean				
	Trash is not overflowing				
	Area is uncluttered				
	If appropriate, supplies for respiratory hygiene are available and posted instructions in place				

C= compliance   NI= needs improvement   NA= not applicable

OTHER STANDARDS RELATED TO IC

Figure 12.1 — INFECTION CONTROL ROUNDS (CONT.)

CRITERIA	REQUIREMENTS	RATING C	NI	N/A	ACTION NEEDED:
Public bathrooms	All surfaces are clean				
	Handwashing supplies are available				
	Trash is not overflowing				
	If cleaning checklist is used, appropriately signed off				
Laboratory	Horizontal and vertical surfaces are clean				
	Biomedical waste is handled per policy				
	PPE is used as needed and per policy				
	Hand hygiene policies are followed				
Pharmacy	Horizontal and vertical surfaces are clean				
	Hoods are maintained per policy				
	Hand hygiene policies are followed				
	Equipment is clean				
	Medication labeling and expiration practices are appropriate				

C= compliance   NI= needs improvement   NA= not applicable

Infection Control Compliance Guide: Understanding the JCAHO's Standards

Figure 12.2   CONSTRUCTION AND RENOVATION IN THE HEALTHCARE FACILITY—
INFECTION CONTROL MEASURES

PURPOSE:

To encourage use of current CDC guidelines in construction and renovation projects in hospitals.

Abbreviations:

ICRA—Infection control risk assessment

PE—Protective environment

ACH—Air changes per hour

HVAC—Heating, ventilation, air conditioning

POLICY:

The facility will do the following:

- Establish a multidisciplinary team that includes infection-control staff to coordinate demolition, construction, and renovation projects and to consider proactive preventive measures at the inception; produce and maintain summary statements of the team's activities.

- Educate both the construction team and healthcare staff in immunocompromised patient-care areas regarding the airborne infection risks associated with construction projects, dispersal of fungal spores during such activities, and methods to control the dissemination of fungal spores.

- Incorporate mandatory adherence agreements for infection control into construction contracts, with penalties for noncompliance and mechanisms to ensure timely correction of problems.

- Establish and maintain surveillance for airborne environmental disease (e.g., aspergillosis) as appropriate during construction, renovation, repair, and demolition activities to ensure the health and safety of immunocompromised patients.

    A. Using active surveillance, monitor for airborne infections in immunocompromised patients.

    B. Periodically review the facility's microbiologic, histopathologic, and postmortem data to identify additional cases.

    C. If cases of aspergillosis or other healthcare-associated airborne fungal infections occur, aggressively pursue the diagnosis with tissue biopsies and cultures as feasible.

- Implement infection-control measures relevant to construction, renovation, maintenance, demolition, and repair.

    A. Before the project gets under way, perform an ICRA to define the scope of the activity and the need for barrier measures.

        1. Determine whether immunocompromised patients may be at risk for exposure to fungal spores from dust generated during the project.

        2. Develop a contingency plan to prevent such exposures.

    B. Implement infection-control measures for external demolition and construction activities.

> **Figure 12.2** — **CONSTRUCTION AND RENOVATION IN THE HEALTHCARE FACILITY—INFECTION CONTROL MEASURES (CONT.)**
>
> 1. Determine if the facility can operate temporarily on recirculated air; if feasible, seal off adjacent air intakes.
> 2. If this is not possible or practical, check the low-efficiency (roughing) filter banks frequently and replace as needed to avoid buildup of particulates.
> 3. Seal windows and reduce wherever possible other sources of outside air intrusion (e.g., open doors in stairwells and corridors).
>
> C. Avoid damaging the underground water system (i.e., buried pipes) to prevent soil and dust contamination of the water.
>
> D. Implement infection-control measures for internal construction activities:
>
> 1. Construct barriers to prevent dust from construction areas from entering patient-care areas; ensure that barriers are impermeable to fungal spores and in compliance with local fire codes.
> 2. Seal off and block return air vents if rigid barriers are used for containment.
> 3. Implement dust-control measures on surfaces and divert pedestrian traffic away from work zones.
> 4. Relocate patients whose rooms are adjacent to work zones depending on their immune status, the scope of the project, the potential for generation of dust or water aerosols, and the methods used to control these aerosols.
>
> E. Perform those engineering and work-site related infection-control measures as needed for internal construction, repairs, and renovations:
>
> 1. Ensure proper operation of the air-handling system in the affected area after erection of barriers and before the room or area is set to negative pressure.
> 2. Create and maintain negative air pressure in work zones adjacent to patient-care areas and ensure that required engineering controls are maintained.
> 3. Monitor negative airflow inside rigid barriers.
> 4. Monitor barriers and ensure integrity of the construction barriers; repair gaps or breaks in barrier joints.
> 5. Seal windows in work zones, if practical; use window chutes for disposal of large pieces of debris as needed, but ensure that the negative pressure differential for the area is maintained.
> 6. Direct pedestrian traffic from construction zones away from patient-care areas to minimize dispersion of dust.
> 7. Provide construction crews with 1) designated entrances, corridors, and elevators wherever practical; 2) essential services (e.g., toilet facilities) and convenience services (e.g., vending machines); 3) protective clothing (e.g., coveralls, footgear, and headgear) for travel to patient-care areas; and 4) a space or anteroom for changing

> **Figure 12.2** — CONSTRUCTION AND RENOVATION IN THE HEALTHCARE FACILITY—
> INFECTION CONTROL MEASURES (CONT.)

>   clothing and storing equipment.
>
>   8. Clean work zones and their entrances daily by 1) wet-wiping tools and tool carts before their removal from the work zone; 2) placing mats with tacky surfaces inside the entrance; and 3) covering debris and securing this covering before removing debris from the work zone.
>
>   9. In patient-care areas, for major repairs that include removal of ceiling tiles and disruption of the space above the false ceiling, use plastic sheets or prefabricated plastic units to contain dust; use a negative pressure system within this enclosure to remove dust; and either pass air through an industrial grade, portable HEPA filter capable of filtration rates of 300 ft^3/min–800 ft^3/min. or exhaust air directly to the outside.
>
>   10. Upon completion of the project, clean the work zone according to facility procedures, and install barrier curtains to contain dust and debris before removing rigid barriers.
>
>   11. Flush the water system to clear sediment from pipes to minimize waterborne microorganism proliferation.
>
>   12. Restore appropriate ACH, humidity, and pressure differential; clean or replace air filters; dispose of spent filters.
>
> - Use airborne-particle sampling as a tool to evaluate barrier integrity.
> - Commission the HVAC system for newly constructed healthcare facilities and renovated spaces before occupancy and use, with emphasis on ensuring proper ventilation for operating rooms, AII rooms, and PE areas.
> - No recommendation is offered regarding routine microbiologic air sampling before, during, or after construction, or before or during occupancy of areas housing immunocompromised patients.
> - If a case of healthcare-acquired aspergillosis or other opportunistic airborne fungal disease occurs during or immediately after construction, implement appropriate follow-up measures.
>
>   A. Review pressure-differential monitoring documentation to verify that pressure differentials in the construction zone and in PE rooms are appropriate for their settings.
>
>   B. Implement corrective engineering measures to restore proper pressure differentials as needed.
>
>   C. Conduct a prospective search for additional cases and intensify retrospective epidemiologic review of the hospital's medical and laboratory records.
>
>   D. If no epidemiologic evidence of ongoing transmission exists, continue routine maintenance in the area to prevent healthcare-acquired fungal disease.

> **Figure 12.2** — **CONSTRUCTION AND RENOVATION IN THE HEALTHCARE FACILITY—INFECTION CONTROL MEASURES (CONT.)**

- If no epidemiologic evidence exists of ongoing transmission of fungal disease, conduct an environmental assessment to find and eliminate the source.

  A. Collect environmental samples from potential sources of airborne fungal spores, preferably by using a high-volume air sampler rather than settle plates.

  B. If either an environmental source of airborne fungi or an engineering problem with filtration or pressure differentials is identified, promptly perform corrective measures to eliminate the source and route of entry.

  C. Use an EPA-registered antifungal biocide (e.g., copper-8-quinolinolate) for decontaminating structural materials.

  D. If an environmental source of airborne fungi is not identified, review infection-control measures, including engineering controls, to identify potential areas for correction or improvement.

  E. If possible, perform molecular subtyping of Aspergillus spp. isolated from patients and the environment to compare their strain identities.

- If air-supply systems to high-risk areas (e.g., PE rooms) are not optimal, use portable, industrial-grade HEPA filters on a temporary basis until rooms with optimal air-handling systems become available.

Source: HcPro, Infection Control Manual for Hospitals, 2004

Chapter Thirteen

Designing a plan for JCAHO survey readiness

This chapter assists you in designing a plan for JCAHO survey readiness. It includes a template of the standards and elements of performance that may be used in a mock survey. It also provides tips on general survey preparation and surveyor interaction.

Take the following steps to facilitate compliance with the JCAHO standards:

1. Study the standards, rationale, and elements of performance.
2. Conduct a self-assessment of current compliance.
3. Develop a detailed to-do list to obtain compliance with all standards (see Figure 1.1 at the end of Chapter 1 for an example of a to-do list).
4. Put in place follow-up actions identified in the to-do list.
5. Reassess compliance with the standards.
6. Revise the to-do list for any areas still needing improvement.
7. Put into practice the additional actions noted in the to-do list.
8. Initiate a mock survey of the IC program and review compliance with the standards. Knowledgeable, objective reviewers should conduct the mock survey (see Figure 13.1 at the end of this chapter for a sample checklist to use in a mock survey).
9. Take actions related to any areas needing improvement the mock survey identifies.
10. Share your excellent program with JCAHO surveyors!

Mock survey

This chapter focuses on step number 8: the mock survey. Its purpose is to mimic the JCAHO survey and objectively access and score your compliance with the standards.

Chapter Thirteen

To achieve this goal, have knowledgeable, objective persons from outside the IC department conduct the review. The IC department will have already completed a self-assessment of its compliance with the standards and implemented actions to improve compliance. Then, once you complete the mock survey and identify areas for improvement, have staff take the steps necessary to achieve compliance. Establish a target date for obtaining compliance.

Use the form in Figure 13.1 on page 117 to assist you in conducting a mock survey for the IC standards and elements of performance. As you complete the mock survey, keep in mind the timeframes necessary for full compliance (see Chapter fourteen of this book for information on scoring guidelines).

Figure 13.1 — INFECTION CONTROL READINESS FOR JCAHO SURVEY

Standard and elements of performance	Responsible person	Date by which to be in compliance	Date of committee approval–if needed
Standard IC.1.10: The risk of development of a healthcare-associated infection (HAI) is minimized through an organization-wide infection control program.			
Elements of performance for IC.1.10			
1. An organization-wide IC program is implemented.			
2. Individuals and/or positions with the authority to take steps to prevent or control the acquisition and transmission of infectious agents are identified.			
3. All applicable organization components and functions are integrated into the IC program.			
4. Systems are in place to communicate with licensed independent practitioners (LIPs), staff, students/trainees, volunteers, and, as appropriate, visitors and patients about infection prevention and control issues, including their responsibilities in preventing the spread of infection within the hospital.			
5. The hospital has systems for reporting identified infections to the following: • Appropriate staff within the hospital • Federal, state, and local public health authorities in accordance with law and regulation • Accrediting bodies (see Sentinel Event Reporting and National Patient Safety Goals) • The referring or receiving organization when a patient was transferred or referred and the presence of an HAI was not known at the time of referral			
6. Systems for investigating outbreaks of infectious diseases are in place.			
7. Applicable policies and procedures are in place throughout the hospital.			
8. Not applicable.			
9. The hospital has a written IC plan that includes the following: • A description of prioritized risks • A statement of the goals of the IC program • A description of the hospital's strategies to minimize, reduce, or eliminate the prioritized risks • A description of how the strategies will be evaluated			

Figure 13.1 — INFECTION CONTROL READINESS FOR JCAHO SURVEY (CONT.)

Standard and elements of performance	Responsible person	Date by which to be in compliance	Date of committee approval–if needed
Standard IC.2.10: The infection control program identifies risks for the acquisition and transmission of infectious agents on an ongoing basis. **Elements of performance for IC.2.10**			
10. The hospital identifies risks for the transmission and acquisition of infectious agents throughout the hospital based on the following factors: • The geographic location and community environment of the hospital, services provided, and characteristics of the population served • The results of the analysis of the hospital's infection prevention and control data • The care, treatment, and services provided			
a. The risk analysis is formally reviewed at least annually and whenever significant changes occur in any of the above factors.			
b. Surveillance activities are used to identify infection prevention and control risks pertaining to the following: • Patients • LIPs, staff, volunteers, and students/trainees • Visitors, as warranted			
Standard IC.3.10: Based on the risks, the hospital establishes priorities and sets goals for preventing the development of healthcare-associated infections within the hospital. **Elements of performance for IC.3.10**			
11. Priorities are established and goals related to preventing the acquisition and transmission of potentially infectious agents are developed, based on the risks identified. These goals include, but are not limited to, the following:			
a. Limiting unprotected exposure to pathogens throughout the hospital.			
b. Enhancing hand hygiene.			
c. Note: This element of performance is currently in field review. It will be provided in a future update as soon as it has been approved. Please refer to Joint Commission Perspectives for more information about this standard.			
d. Minimizing the risk of transmission of infections associated with the use of procedures, medical equipment, and medical devices.			

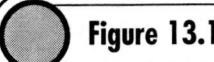

Figure 13.1 — INFECTION CONTROL READINESS FOR JCAHO SURVEY (CONT.)

Standard and elements of performance	Responsible person	Date by which to be in compliance	Date of committee approval–if needed
Standard IC.4.10: Once the hospital has prioritized its goals, strategies must be implemented to achieve the goals **Elements of performance for IC.4.10**			

12. Interventions are designed to incorporate relevant guidelines for infection prevention and control activities.
 	
 Interventions, which include the following, are implemented:
 	
 • An organization-wide hand hygiene program that complies with current CDC hand hygiene guidelines (National Patient Safety Goal #7, requirement #7.a)
 	
 • Methods to reduce the risks associated with procedures, medical equipment, and medical devices including the following:
 	
     – Appropriate storage, cleaning, disinfection, sterilization, and/or disposal of supplies and equipment
 	
     – Reuse of equipment designated by the manufacturer as disposable in a manner that is consistent with regulatory and professional standards
 	
     – The appropriate use of personal protective equipment
 	
 • Implementation of applicable precautions as appropriate are based on the following:
 	
     – The potential for transmission
 	
     – The mechanism of transmission
 	
     – The care setting
 	
     – The emergence and reemergence of pathogens in the community that could affect the hospital
 	
 • Screening for exposure/immunity to infectious diseases with which LIPs, staff, student/trainees, and volunteers may come in contact with in their work is available, as warranted
 	
 • Referral for assessment, potential testing, immunization and/or prophylaxis/treatment, and counseling as appropriate of LIPs, staff, students/trainees, and volunteers who are identified as potentially having an infectious disease or risk of infectious disease that may put the population they serve at risk
 	
 • Referral for assessment, potential testing, immunization and/or prophylaxis/treatment, and counseling as appropriate of patients, students/trainees, and volunteers who have been exposed to infectious disease(s) at the hospital and LIPs or staff who are occupationally exposed
 	
 • Reduction of risks associated with animals brought into the hospital			

Chapter Thirteen

Figure 13.1 — INFECTION CONTROL READINESS FOR JCAHO SURVEY (CONT.)

Standard and elements of performance	Responsible person	Date by which to be in compliance	Date of committee approval–if needed
Standard IC.5.10: The infection control program evaluates the effectiveness of the infection control interventions and, as necessary, redesigns the infection control interventions. **Elements of performance for IC.5.10**			
13. The hospital formally evaluates and revises the goals and program (or portions of the program) at least annually and whenever risks are significantly changed.			
a. The evaluation addresses changes in the scope of the IC program (for example, resulting from the introduction of new services or new sites of care).			
b. The evaluation addresses changes in the results of the IC program risk analysis.			
c. The evaluation addresses emerging and reemerging problems in the healthcare community that potentially affect the hospital (e.g., highly infectious agents).			
d. The evaluation addresses the assessment of the success or failure of interventions for preventing and controlling infection.			
e. The evaluation addresses responses to concerns raised by leadership and others within the hospital.			
f. The evaluation addresses the evolution of relevant infection prevention and control guidelines that are based on evidence or, in the absence of evidence, expert consensus.			
Standard IC.6.10: As part of emergency management activities, the organization prepares to respond to an influx, or the risk of an influx, of infectious patients. **Elements of performance for IC.6.10**			
14. The organization plans its response to an influx or risk of an influx of infectious patients.			
a. The organization has a plan for managing an influx of potentially infectious patients/residents/clients over an extended period of time.			
b. The organization • determines how it will keep abreast of current information about the emergence of epidemics or new infections that may result in the organization activating its response • determines how it will disseminate critical information to staff and other key practitioners • identifies resources in the community (through local, state, and/or federal public health systems) for obtaining additional information			

| Figure 13.1 | INFECTION CONTROL READINESS FOR JCAHO SURVEY (CONT.) |

Standard and elements of performance	Responsible person	Date by which to be in compliance	Date of committee approval–if needed
Standard IC.7.10: The infection control program is managed effectively. **Elements of performance for IC.7.10**			
15. The hospital assigns responsibility for managing IC program activities to one or more individuals whose number, competency, and skill mix are determined by the goals and objectives of the IC activities.			
a. Qualification of the individual(s) responsible for managing the IC program are determined by the risks entailed in the services provided, the hospital's patient population(s), and the complexity of the activities that will be carried out. Note: Qualifications may be met through ongoing education, training, experience, and/or certification (such as that offered by the Certification Board for Infection Control [CBIC] in the prevention and control of infections).			
b. This individual(s) coordinates all infection prevention and control within the hospital.			
c. This individual(s) facilitates ongoing monitoring of the effectiveness of prevention and/or control activities and interventions.			

Chapter Thirteen

Figure 13.1 INFECTION CONTROL READINESS FOR JCAHO SURVEY (CONT.)

Standard and elements of performance	Responsible person	Date by which to be in compliance	Date of committee approval–if needed
Standard IC.8.10: Representatives from relevant components/functions within the hospital collaborate to implement the infection control program. **Elements of performance for IC.8.10**			
16. Hospital leaders including medical staff, LIPs, and other direct and indirect patient-care staff (including, when applicable, pharmacy, laboratory, administration, central supply/sterilization services, housekeeping, building maintenance/engineering, and food services) collaborate on an ongoing basis with the qualified individual(s) managing the IC program.			
a. These representatives participate in the following: • Development of strategies for each component's/function's role in the IC program • Assessment of the adequacy of the human, information, physical, and financial resources allocated to support infection prevention and control activities • Assessment of the overall failure or success of key processes for preventing and controlling infection • The review and revision of the IC program as warranted to improve outcomes			
Standard IC.9.10: Hospital leaders allocate adequate resources for the infection control program. **Elements of performance for IC.9.10**			
17. Leaders review on an ongoing basis (but no less frequently than annually) the effectiveness of the hospital's infection prevention and control activities and report their findings to the integrated patient safety program.			
a. Adequate systems to access information are provided to support infection prevention and control activities.			
b. When applicable, adequate laboratory support is provided to support infection prevention and control activities.			
c. Adequate equipment and supplies are provided to support infection prevention and control activities.			

Chapter Fourteen

Scoring guidelines: How to make sure you're successful

This chapter provides you with the Joint Commission on Accreditation of Healthcare Organizations' (JCAHO) scoring guidelines for the infection control (IC) standards and for the elements of performance (EP) for each standard. These scoring guidelines should assist you in confirming your organization's preparedness to meet the IC standards.

All students want to know two things: how strict the teacher is and how the test will be scored. In the case of a JCAHO survey, the "teacher"—i.e., the surveyor—and his or her interpretations can vary. But if you know the scoring methods, you will ensure that you are prepared and can defend your interpretation of all of the JCAHO standards.

Designing a strategy to ensure a compliant score

The JCAHO made the 2005 standards much more detailed than earlier versions—and much more concise. EPs provide better guidance on how to ensure that your organization is compliant with their intent. Where the standard and its EP are not sufficiently clear, the JCAHO provides a statement of rationale to further define what compliance with the standard means for your organization. The more detail the JCAHO provides, the better the chance that facilities will actually meet the intent of the standard.

Information to help your organization become compliant with the JCAHO IC standards is divided into the following three groups:

1. Standard: A statement of the expected performance and the structures or processes required for an organization to provide safe, high quality care. An organization's compliance or noncompliance with a standard is noted by checking the appropriate box in the margin by the standard. Accreditation decisions are based on simple counts of noncompliance with standards.

Chapter Fourteen

2. Rationale: A statement of background, justification, or additional information for a standard. A standard's rationale is not scored. Because the rationale for a standard is sometimes self-evident, not every standard has one written.

3. EPs: The specific performance expectation and the structures or processes required for an organization to provide safe, high quality care. EP scoring determines a hospital's overall compliance with a standard. Scores are as follows (see Figures 14.1–14.4):

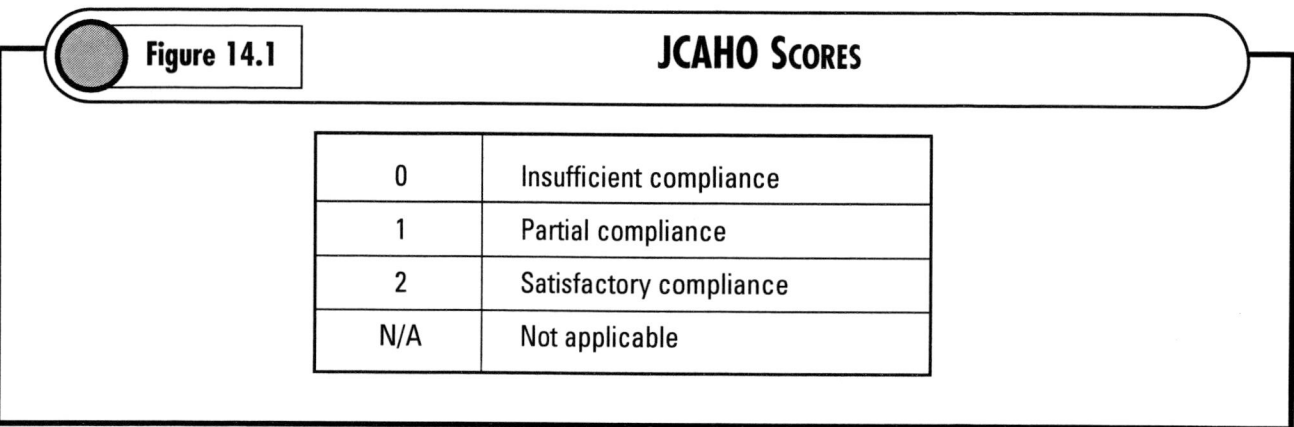

Figure 14.1 JCAHO Scores

0	Insufficient compliance
1	Partial compliance
2	Satisfactory compliance
N/A	Not applicable

You will find a measure-of-success icon next to some EPs. A measure of success needs to be developed when an organization is found, through either the periodic performance review or the onsite surveys, to be out of compliance with a standard. A measure of success is a quantifiable means of determining whether an action has been effective and is being sustained.

Scoring categories

The EPs for standards will be scored in three categories—A, B, and C—based on two factors:

1. Validation that your organization is in compliance with the EP
2. The length of time it has been in compliance

Category A

Category A evaluates whether EPs related to infrastructure for safe IC practices (e.g., procedures, documentation tools) have been implemented. The requirement will normally be scored as a 0 or 2; however, a score of 1 is possible if the length of time that your organization has had this practice in place is insufficient to warrant a rating of 2. Your organization's compliance will be scored in accordance with the following length of that EP's practice in your institution:

Figure 14.2 — Compliance Timeframes for Category A EPs

SCORE	INITIAL SURVEY	FULL SURVEY
2	Four months or more	12 months or more
1	Two to three months	Six to 11 months
0	Fewer than two months	Fewer than six months

Category B

Category B EPs also have an infrastructure element, but they will be evaluated on the basis of a qualitative component as well. These EPs also are commonly scored 0 or 2, unless the quality, adequacy, or completeness of compliance is not self-evident. If your organization falls into the latter assessment of compliance, a score of 1 is possible. If your organization's actions in complying with a Category B EP are not easily documented, your organization will need to demonstrate that it meets the intent of the EP by following "principles of good process design." Good process design

- is consistent with the organization's mission, values, and goals
- meets defined needs of patients
- reflects current standards of care
- integrates safety information and knowledge (e.g., system changes due to internal and external safety information)
- incorporates actions that have been shown to meet EPs through relevant performance improvement results
- meets all components of EPs as documented by the JCAHO

You only need to demonstrate performance for all EPs in Category B if JCAHO surveyors question the quality, adequacy, or comprehensiveness of compliance.

Again, your organization's compliance with EP requirements will be scored on the basis of a documented track record as follows:

Chapter Fourteen

> **Figure 14.3** — **COMPLIANCE TIMEFRAMES FOR CATEGORY B EPs**
>
> | SCORE | INITIAL SURVEY | FULL SURVEY |
> |---|---|---|
> | 2 | Four months or more | 12 months or more |
> | 1 | Two to three months | Six to 11 months |
> | 0 | Fewer than two months | Fewer than six months |

To determine your organization's score for EPs in this category, the following guidelines apply:

- Your EP score is 2 if your organization considered all applicable principles of the standards and meets the track-record achievements for score 2
- Your EP score is 1 if your organization considered only some of the applicable principles and/or meets the preceding track-record achievements for score 1
- Your EP score is 0 if your organization did not consider any of the applicable principles and/or meets the track-record achievements for score 0

Category C

Category C EPs are scored on the basis of the number of times your organization doesn't perform to the principles of the standard. They may be scored 0, 1, or 2, depending on the number of times your organization fails to meet the standard's principles:

- Your score will be EP 2 if there is no or one instance of noncompliance with an EP and your organization meets the track-record achievements for score 2.
- Your score will be EP 1 if there are two instances of noncompliance with an EP and your organization meets the track-record achievements for score 1.
- Your score will be EP 0 if there are three or more instances of noncompliance with an EP and your organization meets the track-record achievements for score 0.

The following documented compliance track record is used to judge compliance with EPs:

Figure 14.4 — COMPLIANCE TIMEFRAMES FOR CATEGORY C EPs

SCORE	INITIAL SURVEY	FULL SURVEY
2	Four months or more	12 months or more
1	Two to three months	Six to 11 months
0	Fewer than two months	Fewer than six months

Compliance with the standard

Now that you have evaluated your performance in meeting EPs, you can determine your compliance with the standard itself:

- Your hospital is not in compliance with the standard if any EP is scored 0
- Your hospital is in compliance with a standard if 65% or more of the standard's EPs are scored 2

See Figure 14.5 on page 128 for a recap of the IC standards and their EPs as specified by the JCAHO.

CHAPTER FOURTEEN

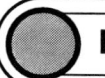

Figure 14.5 — IC STANDARDS, EPs, AND HOW EPS ARE CATEGORIZED

IC standards, EPs, and how EPs are categorized

In the table below, you will find a recap of the IC standards and their EPs as specified by the JCAHO. The exact wording of the JCAHO standards and their EPs should be checked in the standards, as only the JCAHO number for the EP is listed. The table allows you to quickly identify the scoring category for each EP, assess your performance for each EP, and determine whether your organization is compliant with the standard.

Standard and Element of Performance	EPs Category	Measure of success icon	Score (0, 1, 2, NA)
IC.1.10 An organization-wide IC program is implemented.	NA	NA	Compliant? Yes or No
1	B		
2	B		
3	B		
4	B		
5	B		
6	B		
7	B		
8	N/A		
9	B		
IC.2.10 The IC program identifies risks for the acquisition and transmission of infectious agents on an ongoing basis.	NA	NA	Compliant? Yes or No
1	B		
2	A		
3	B		
IC.3.10 Based on risks, the hospital establishes priorities and sets goals for preventing the development of healthcare-associated infections within the hospital.	NA	NA	Compliant? Yes or No
1	B		
2	A		
3	A		
4 *In field review*			
5	A		
IC.4.10 The hospital plans and implements interventions to address the IC issues that it finds important based on prioritized risks and associated surveillance data.	NA	NA	Compliant? Yes or No
1	B		
2	C	√	
3	C	√	
4	B		

SCORING GUIDELINES: HOW TO MAKE SURE YOU'RE SUCCESSFUL

Figure 14.5 — **IC STANDARDS, EPs, AND HOW EPS ARE CATEGORIZED (CONT.)**

Standard and Element of Performance	EPs Category	Measure of success icon	Score (0, 1, 2, NA)
5	C	√	
6	C		
7	C		
8	B		
IC.5.10 The IC program evaluates the effectiveness of the IC interventions and, as necessary, redesigns the IC interventions.	NA	NA	Compliant? Yes or No
1	A		
2	B		
3	B		
4	B		
5	B		
6	B		
7	B		
IC.6.10 As part of emergency management activities, the organization prepares to respond to an influx, or the risk of an influx, of infectious patients.	NA	NA	Compliant? Yes or No
1			
2			
3			
IC.7.10 The IC program is managed effectively.	NA	NA	Compliant? Yes or No
1	B		
2	B		
3	B		
4	B		
IC.8.10 Representatives from relevant components/functions within the hospital collaborate to implement the IC program.	NA	NA	Compliant? Yes or No
1	B		
2	B		
IC.9.10 Hospital leaders allocate adequate resources for the IC program.	NA	NA	Compliant? Yes or No
1	A		
2	B		
3	B		
4	B		

Using the files on your *Infection Control Compliance Guide: Understanding the JCAHO's Standards* CD-ROM

The following is a list of file names and a brief description of the documents contained on this book's CD-ROM:

File name	Document
README.doc	Instructions on using the CD-ROM
Observe.doc	Hand-hygiene observation tool
Hpolicy.doc	Hand-hygiene policy
Rounds.doc	IC compliance rounds
Policy.doc	Construction policy
Mock.doc	Mock survey form
EPcat.doc	Categories of EPs
Risk.doc	IC risk assessment
ICcomp.doc	IC competency assessment
Resource.doc	IC resources
ToDo.doc	IC compliance to-do list
BBform.doc	Bloodborne pathogen post-exposure form
CDC.doc	CDC hand-hygiene recommendations
CDC1.doc	CDC hand-hygiene guidelines fact sheet

To run the *Infection Control Compliance Guide: Understanding the JCAHO's Standards* CD-ROM, take the following steps:

1. Insert the CD-ROM into your CD-ROM drive.
2. Double-click on the "My Computer" icon, next double-click on the CD drive icon.
3. Double-click on the files you wish to open.
4. To save a file to your facility's system, click on "File," then "Save as," and select the location where you wish to save the file and then click "Save."